EATING FOR GASTROPARESIS:
Guidelines, Tips & Recipes

By Crystal Zaborowski Saltrelli
Certified Health Coach, AADP

Author's Note

The information contained in this book is for educational purposes only. It is not intended or implied to be a substitute for professional medical advice, diagnosis, or treatment. You should always consult your doctor or qualified healthcare provider to determine the appropriateness of the information for your own situation and for guidance regarding your medical condition and treatment plan.

Contents

INTRODUCTION

I'd like to congratulate you for seeking out and purchasing this book. Making the decision to be proactive about managing gastroparesis (GP) is the first step in learning to live (well!) with the condition.

I was diagnosed with idiopathic gastroparesis over a decade ago at the age of 23. Between the one-page dietary handout I was given by my doctor and the information I found online in the days and weeks afterward, I quickly whittled my diet down to a handful of low-fat, low-fiber staples.

I struggled with constant and often debilitating digestive symptoms. I visited doctor after doctor, traveling thousands of miles to the best medical centers in the country. I didn't receive the answers I was looking for, but I did begin to receive additional diagnoses, including colonic inertia, iron deficiency anemia, orthostatic hypotension, polycystic ovarian syndrome, and Reynaud's syndrome.

Five years later, despite following the prescribed diet, trying all of the available drugs, enduring countless tests, and seeking out alternative practitioners, I was no better off. I'd lost nearly 50 pounds, I was unable to work, unable to sleep, unable to eat, and I'd wracked up a mountain of debt searching for a solution to my worsening health problems.

Fueled by desperation and the belief that there had to be something I could do to get my life back, I enrolled at the Institute for Integrative Nutrition to study holistic health and nutrition. That was a turning point for me and I've since used what I learned to help myself and thousands of others around the world employ dietary, nutritional, and lifestyle changes to ease their gastroparesis symptoms, enhance their quality of life, and improve their overall health and wellbeing.

While there are several other aspects to a successful gastroparesis management plan, I know from both personal and professional experience that the dietary component is often the most confusing. Whether you have gastroparesis yourself or you're caring for someone who does, the information and recipes in this book will help to alleviate the sense of overwhelm and uncertainty that often surrounds a "gastroparesis-friendly" diet. What's more, by following the suggestions in this book, you'll be working toward improving both your digestive function and your overall health, as poor nutrition and declining gut health is a significant risk of the standard "gastroparesis-friendly" diet.

Thanks to the advice laid out here and in my second book, *Living (Well!) with Gastroparesis*, I now feel better than I have in ten years. These days gastroparesis is the least of my challenges as the mother of a healthy, active two-year-old.

Many of my subsequent diagnoses, which I believe were largely due to the chronic stress and poor nutrition of struggling with gastroparesis, have also improved or resolved completely. My intention in writing this book is to help you avoid the dietary mistakes that I made so that you can get to a point of living well much more quickly than I did.

Since I published the first edition of this book in 2010, my knowledge of both gastroparesis and nutrition has expanded dramatically and some of my recommendations have changed. This book represents my current thinking on digestive health and nutrition and encompasses the best advice that I have to offer to those dealing with gastroparesis.

Though some of the suggestions may seem difficult or drastic at first, I have not included anything that I haven't done myself, had success implementing with clients, and truly believe to be beneficial for those who want to live well, and especially for those hoping to get well, following a gastroparesis diagnosis.

As you read, please keep in mind that I am not a physician. The information in this book is based on my training in holistic health and nutrition, my personal journey with gastroparesis, and five years of experience as a Health Coach specializing in gastroparesis management. What I'm offering you are guidelines and suggestions – not medical advice. Dietary tolerances, severity of symptoms, and nutritional considerations vary greatly among those with gastroparesis. Please consult your physician if you have any questions as to whether or not a particular suggestion is appropriate for you.

UNDERSTANDING & MANAGING GASTROPARESIS

Before we get started with a gastroparesis-friendly diet, I'd like to ensure that you have a good understanding of the diagnosis you've received. Misconceptions about gastroparesis and gastroparesis management are common and often lead to unnecessary frustration.

Gastroparesis (GP) means that the stomach empties more slowly than it should. GP is a functional gastrointestinal disorder. There is no structural abnormality or physical obstruction that is causing the stomach to empty too slowly. Rather the problem is caused by the way the stomach *functions*.

While the focus of this book is on dietary strategies for managing gastroparesis, what you eat is only one of many considerations when it comes to alleviating symptoms of the disorder. In fact, dietary modifications alone, especially those that are nutritionally-sound, are unlikely to provide adequate symptom relief.

If you want to live well, and especially if your goal is get well, it is imperative that you carry out the suggestions in this book as *one part* of a comprehensive gastroparesis management plan. In addition to dietary modifications, an effective management plan should include:

- Supportive lifestyle habits, encompassing adequate high-quality sleep, regular mild to moderate physical activity, socializing, and engaging in activities that bring you joy;

- Stress reduction and management, as well as a consistent relaxation practice;

- Complementary therapies, which may consist of supplements, herbal remedies, and/or treatments such as acupuncture, massage, or hypnosis; and,

- Appropriate medical care, which may or may not include prescription drugs, nonprescription drugs, and other interventions.

An attempt to manage gastroparesis solely through dietary changes is unlikely to result in optimum symptom management, quality of life, and long-term health and wellbeing. It *is* likely to result in nutritional deficiencies over time and may contribute to additional health concerns. So do implement what you read in this book, but please do it *as part* of a larger plan.

For more information about building a comprehensive gastroparesis management plan, including free worksheets and videos, please visit the Book Resources page at www.EatingForGastroparesis.com.

PART ONE:
THE GUIDELINES

In this section, we'll cover the basic guidelines of a gastroparesis-friendly (GP-friendly) diet. As you read, remember that you know your body and your boundaries better than anyone else. Some of the suggestions may not be appropriate for you given your symptoms, tolerances, goals, or preferences.

Dietary modifications are a symptom-management tool, not a treatment for gastroparesis itself. This does not mean that gastroparesis does not or cannot get better, of course, just that following the dietary guidelines in this book won't necessarily address the underlying cause of the disorder. In conjunction with the other aspects of a comprehensive management plan, however, dietary changes can significantly alleviate day-to-day symptoms and support the body's natural healing mechanisms.

To date, no studies have been conducted to determine which specific foods or types of foods alleviate or exacerbate symptoms in those with gastroparesis. The standard dietary instructions are based on the basic science of digestion, as well as the experience and observations of patients and clinicians over time. Similarly, the guidelines set forth in this book are based on a combination of my knowledge of nutrition, digestion, and gut health, as well as my personal experience with gastroparesis and several years coaching others with the condition.

10 Guidelines of a Gastroparesis-Friendly Diet

1. Eat smaller meals.

2. Reduce dietary fat.

3. Reduce dietary fiber.

4. Limit foods with indigestible parts.

5. Choose a variety of GP-friendly, nutrient-rich foods.

6. Supplement with nutrient-rich liquids, as necessary.

7. Chew thoroughly.

8. Eat slowly, calmly, and in a relaxed environment.

9. Reduce or eliminate foods that impair gut health, provoke symptoms, and/or compromise digestion.

10. Modify the guidelines according to your symptoms, circumstances, and goals.

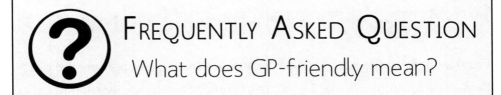

FREQUENTLY ASKED QUESTION
What does GP-friendly mean?

Throughout this book, you'll see the term "GP-friendly" used to describe foods and recipes. When I use that term, I'm indicating that:

- it's relatively low in fat, low in fiber, and easy to digest.
- it doesn't contain whole nuts, seeds, skins, hulls, peels, dried fruit, raw vegetables, or other food with indigestible parts.
- it's generally supportive of overall health, including gut health.
- it's likely to be well-tolerated by many people with gastroparesis.

Anything that meets these criteria is unlikely to cause any serious problems. The catch? There are things that I consider "GP-friendly" that don't agree with me personally. Likewise, there may be some that don't agree with you.

As I tell my clients, GP-friendly doesn't always mean <your name here>-friendly. While I know that can be frustrating and it's tempting to stick to a handful of "safe" foods, I encourage you to continue experimenting — particularly with things that *are* GP-friendly — for the sake of your overall nutrition, as well as your sanity.

Also keep in mind that eating foods that you do not tolerate, even those that are not GP-friendly, may provoke symptoms in the short-term but will not further delay gastric emptying in the long term or make your gastroparesis more severe overall.

Modify the Guidelines According to Your Symptoms, Circumstances, and Goals

I'm starting with the last guideline because it's the most important and often the most frustrating. While I wish that I could tell you exactly what to eat, the unfortunate truth is this: there is no single "gastroparesis diet." In fact, you'd be hard-pressed to find even a single food that's well-tolerated by each and every person with gastroparesis. Instead, foods tend to fall along a spectrum from "generally well-tolerated" to "likely to aggravate symptoms."

Why do tolerances vary so much from person to person? There are several possibilities. One factor may be the many different causes of gastroparesis, including viral infections, abdominal surgery, physical or emotional trauma, anorexia nervosa, diabetes, and several other underlying medical conditions.

There are many people with gastroparesis that also have other digestive issues, such as Irritable Bowel Syndrome, gallbladder disease (or gallbladder removal), chronic constipation, Celiac disease, lactose intolerance, fructose malabsorption, small intestinal bacterial overgrowth, and/or food allergies. Others may have additional health considerations, such as autoimmune disorders, neurological issues, or cardiac disease, which also require specific dietary intervention.

In addition, the actual rate at which the stomach empties varies greatly among those diagnosed with gastroparesis, from mildly delayed to severely delayed. What's more, the severity of one's symptoms does not always correlate to the severity of the delay in gastric emptying.

Given all of these variables, it makes sense that the specifics of a gastroparesis-friendly diet may differ from person to person. Dietary choices are further complicated by the fact that symptoms tend to ebb and flow. Individual tolerances may vary from week to week or even from day to day.

Whether a particular food or meal will exacerbate symptoms can depend on portion size, how quickly it's eaten, whether there's anxiety around eating, and what was eaten earlier that day or even the day before. Symptoms may also be influenced by overall stress levels, fluctuations in hormones, lack of sleep, or other lifestyle factors.

The bottom line is this: there is no one-size-fits-all diet for gastroparesis. But there are a set of effective guidelines from which you can develop your *own* gastroparesis-friendly diet. Careful trial-and-error – within the boundaries of these general guidelines — is the best way to figure out exactly what works for you. Throughout the remainder of the book, I'll provide you with ideas, suggestions, and guidance but it's your responsibility to tailor the specifics to your unique circumstances.

Eat Smaller Meals

Decreasing meal size can alleviate the fullness, distention, and pain that those with gastroparesis often experience after eating, as well as help the stomach to empty more quickly. In fact, one of the primary determinants of gastric emptying time in a normally functioning stomach is the volume of food ingested. A larger meal will generally take longer to empty than a smaller meal.

For those with gastroparesis, a good rule of thumb is to eat about one-half of a "normal" sized meal. These days it can be hard to determine what constitutes a normal-sized meal, so a more helpful suggestion might be to consume around one-and-one-half (1-1/2) cups of food per meal. Depending on exactly how much food you can tolerate at one time and how many hours you sleep, you may need to eat four, five, or even six meals per day, waiting

? FREQUENTLY ASKED QUESTION
What constitutes a small meal?

When eating small meals throughout the day, it's easy to get into a snacking mind-set, opting for single foods, like crackers, cereal, or a banana, rather than well-balanced meals.

While this might be the easiest way to go, it's not optimal for nutrition or satisfaction. As much as possible, all meals should be well-balanced with appropriate portions of nutrient-rich, GP-friendly carbohydrates and protein, as well as a small amount of healthy fat. It should look like a "regular" meal... only smaller.

The meals don't have to be particularly complicated. For example:
- 2 eggs, scrambled; 1/2 cup cantaloupe
- 1-1/2 cups Chicken & Root Vegetable soup (page 116)
- 3 oz salmon; ½ cup white rice; ½ cup cooked carrots

High-quality nutritional supplement drinks (see page 30) or home-made smoothies may be used as a meal replacement, so long as they include adequate amounts of fat and protein. Adding a tablespoon of nut butter and a scoop of protein powder or Great Lakes Unflavored Kosher gelatin to a fruit smoothie, for example, can turn it from a mostly-carbohydrate snack into a well-balanced meal replacement.

Eating well-balanced meals throughout the day will help to optimize nutrition, reduce cravings, increase satisfaction, enhance energy, and stabilize blood sugar (this is important for everyone, not just diabetics).

two-and-half to three hours between each one.

Some may tolerate four slightly larger meals, some may do better with six slightly smaller meals, but grazing or snacking all day isn't recommended.

Grazing often adds up to a larger quantity of food than defined meals and may increase fullness and other GP symptoms, especially in the evening and throughout the night. Grazing also prevents the cleansing waves that occur throughout the intestines between meals. This makes it easier for bacteria to grow up into the small intestine causing additional symptoms and possibly even food intolerances.

You may find that you can tolerate larger meals in the morning but need to reduce meal size as the day goes on. Likewise, you may tolerate more solid foods earlier in the day and feel better eating soft foods or drinking nutrient-rich liquids in the evening. On the other hand, if your symptoms tend to be worse in the morning, you may need to start the day with liquids or soft foods and switch to small meals later on.

Experiment with various meal sizes, compositions, and schedules to see which combination works best for you. Ideally, you want to find the point at which you're experiencing fewer symptoms, but still consuming regular meals that contain adequate calories and well-balanced nutrition. Again, keep in mind that your diet is only one of several ways to improve symptom management but it is the only way to provide your body with the nutrition that it needs to function properly.

If this experimentation seems like an arduous task, take it one step at a time. First, invest in a small notebook that you can use as a food journal (see page 21). Then, for one week try eating a well-balanced mini-meal consisting of about one and a half cups of food every three hours. For most people this will result in five small meals per day. Keep track of how you feel.

From there, tailor your schedule and pattern based on your experience. For example:

- If you experience fullness throughout the day, try reducing your meal size and increasing your meal frequency. This will likely result in six small meals (about 1 to 1-1/4 cups of food), each about two and a half hours apart.

- If you find that you're hungry before three hours passes, try increasing your meal size slightly and/or increasing the amount of protein and fat in your meals within the GP-friendly guidelines.

- If you experience more fullness in the evening or first thing in morning, try reducing the size of your last two meals and/or focusing on nutrient-rich liquids or soft foods in the afternoon and evening.

- If you find yourself overeating late in the day, try increasing the size of your morning meal(s) and/or focusing on increasing the healthy fat and protein within your tolerances.

Keep in mind that once you figure out which particular way of eating best suits your needs and preferences, you may need to tweak your schedule, meal pattern, and food choices as your symptoms wax and wane over time. Gastroparesis is not a static disorder and you will likely have good days and bad days, especially as you are experimenting. It's important to be flexible and remember that flare-ups will come and go.

As you identify your personal tolerances, establish your comprehensive management plan, and become consistent with your choices, you will almost certainly experience fewer bad days and more consistency overall.

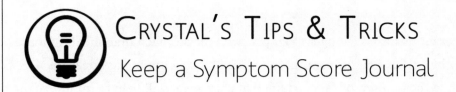

CRYSTAL'S TIPS & TRICKS
Keep a Symptom Score Journal

When first starting out on a gastroparesis-friendly diet a simple food journal can be really helpful. There is often no better way to figure out what does and does not work for you than by consistently keeping track of what you eat and how you feel.

It needn't be time-consuming. You don't need to track calories or other nutritional information. Simply keep a little notebook with you throughout the day to jot down your meals (time, what you ate, and approximate portion sizes) and any symptoms that you experience throughout the day.

It's also helpful to note your general stress level, as well as anything out of the ordinary, such as menstruation, a sleepless night, a new supplement or medication, etc.

At the end of each day, write down a "symptom score" from 1 to 5. One being a great symptom-free day; five being a day full of horrible symptoms. Do this for at least four weeks and watch for patterns that emerge over time between the severity of your symptoms and what, how, and/or how much you eat.

This will also help you to determine how your digestion responds to lifestyle choices, hormonal changes, and other non-dietary factors. With this information, you may be able to tailor your diet to minimize symptom flare-ups related to these factors.

Reduce Dietary Fat

Higher fat meals take longer to empty from the stomach than meals that are lower in fat. This is true for everyone, even those without gastroparesis. Decreasing the amount of fat consumed at each meal will help to minimize the amount of time that meals take to empty from the stomach. For this reason, it's usually helpful for those with gastroparesis to reduce the overall amount of fat in their diet.

A lower-fat diet does not mean a no-fat diet. Fat is an essential nutrient for health, including proper vitamin absorption, brain function, hormonal balance, and blood sugar regulation. Eliminating all fat from the diet is neither appropriate nor necessary, especially in the context of a comprehensive management plan. (Even if you were to eliminate all dietary fat, the stomach would still empty those fat-free meals more slowly than normal due to the underlying gastroparesis.)

Specific fat tolerances vary, but a good starting point for experimentation is around 40 grams of fat per day. Some GPers may find that they do better with closer to 30 grams per day, while others may be able to consume 50 grams without exacerbating symptoms.

It's okay to experiment with eating various amounts of fat from day to day; it will not make your gastroparesis more severe in the long-term. If there is a particular higher-fat food that you tolerate, there is no reason to remove it from your diet unless it begins to provoke symptoms. This is especially true for nutrient-rich sources of fat like the ones mentioned on the following page.

It's best to add a small amount of fat to each meal throughout the day, rather than consuming one high-fat meal. For example, you might eat five meals that have between 6 and 10 grams of fat each.

Some people with gastroparesis find that they tolerate more fat in the morning and less as the day goes on. If that's the case, be careful not to consume so much fat early in the day that you feel too full or sick to eat properly for the rest of the day. If the opposite is true, be weary of eating so much fat in the evening that you wake up full and symptomatic in the morning.

Most sources of fat are considered GP-friendly. You should avoid fried foods and fatty meats, however, as these are especially hard to digest. You should also avoid all trans fats, listed on packaged food as partially hydrogenated oils, and refined vegetables oils, including soy, corn, and canola. These are unstable fats that are not health-promoting and may increase inflammation in all parts of the body, including the digestive tract.

My favorite cooking fats are full-fat butter, ghee (clarified butter), olive oil, red palm oil, and coconut oil. Coconut oil tends to be especially well-tolerated by and beneficial for those with digestive symptoms.

Additional sources of fat in a GP-friendly diet may include nut or seed butters, whole eggs, ground meats, fatty fish, and avocados. With all sources of fat, quantity tends to be the key determinant of how well it's tolerated. Again, slow and careful experimentation is key!

Amount of dietary fat:

- Olive, coconut, and red palm oil – 14 grams per Tbsp
- Butter and ghee – 11 grams per Tbsp
- Salmon – about 10 grams per 3 ounces (varies depending on type)
- Almond butter – 9 grams per Tbsp
- Peanut butter – 8 grams per Tbsp
- Sunflower seed butter – 8 grams per Tbsp
- Avocado - 5 grams per 1/4 cup
- Eggs – 5 grams per egg

Reduce Dietary Fiber

Like fat, fiber increases the gastric emptying time of a meal. Again, this is true for everyone not just those with gastroparesis. Reducing overall fiber in the diet may help to alleviate symptoms of fullness, distention, pain, and bloating.

The amount of fiber tolerated will vary from person to person, but an average total for a gastroparesis-friendly diet is about 12-15 grams of fiber per day. I do not advocate removing all fiber from the diet. As with fat, fiber is necessary for overall health and digestive function, and even removing all fiber from the diet would not result in a normalization of gastric emptying. A very low fiber diet typically relies on processed and refined foods, which may contribute to issues with weight maintenance, blood sugar dysregulation (even in non-diabetics), and bacterial overgrowth.

It is recommended that those with gastroparesis avoid high-fiber, hard-to-digest foods like raw vegetables, most raw fruits, and brown rice. Instead, opt for easier-to-digest and/or lower-fiber versions of these foods, such as well-cooked or juiced vegetables, cooked or pureed fruits, and white rice.

Some moderate-fiber foods, such as gluten-free whole grains or pseudo-grains, aren't associated with bezoar formation and pose no real risk other than potentially exacerbating symptoms in the short-term. If you can eat properly prepared whole grains without becoming too full to meet your caloric and nutrition needs, it's not necessary to completely remove them from your diet. Examples include quinoa, buckwheat, and millet. Soaking these grains for 8-24 hours prior to cooking makes them easier to digest and removes anti-nutrients that impair absorption of vitamins and minerals.

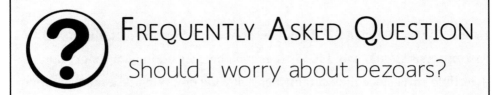

FREQUENTLY ASKED QUESTION
Should I worry about bezoars?

Many GPers worry about bezoars, hardened masses of undigested food that can collect in the stomach causing severe symptoms. Bezoars may need to be removed by a doctor via endoscopy.

Unless your doctor has indicated that you have a high risk of developing a bezoar, the need for concern is low. In fact, bezoars are a fairly rare complication, occurring in only about 20% of the gastroparesis population.

If you also have impaired motility of the small bowel (CIPO), you may be at a higher risk of bezoar formation. Once you've had a bezoar, you are more likely to get another and should take extra precautions, including avoiding all foods listed below.

Foods specifically associated with bezoar formation include: apples, berries, broccoli, Brussels sprouts, coconut (meat not milk), corn, green beans, figs, oranges, persimmons, potato peels, and sauerkraut.

Bulk fiber supplements such as Metamucil, Perdiem, Fibercon and Citrucel should be avoided as they contain insoluble fiber and may exacerbate symptoms and promote bezoar formation.

Limit or Avoid Foods with Indigestible Parts

In addition to reducing the overall amount of fiber in the diet, those with gastroparesis should avoid foods that can't be chewed fully or that contain indigestible parts since they can further delay the emptying of a meal and may contribute to the formation of bezoars. These include broccoli, popcorn, dried fruit, whole nuts and seeds, skins and peels, hulls, legumes, and dried beans.

Ultimately, what you choose to eat or not eat depends on your personal tolerances, physician's advice, severity of symptoms, and comfort level. Some people with gastroparesis regularly eat foods that are not considered GP-friendly without issue. If you'd like to experiment, start with pureed forms of harder-to-digest foods, such as hummus instead of chickpeas or a blueberry smoothie rather than blueberries.

Eat a Variety of Nutrient-Rich GP-friendly Foods

Many gastroparesis-friendly diets rely on a handful of "safe" staples, often white, refined foods. Eating the same foods day after day isn't optimal, as various foods provide different vitamins, minerals, and other necessary nutrients. What's more, eating the same foods every day may increase the risk of developing food sensitivities and bacterial imbalances, especially for those with compromised gut health.

Try to have at least three days worth of meal plans, consisting of a variety of protein, fat, and carbohydrate sources, that you can rotate throughout the week. You'll find a comprehensive list of gastroparesis-friendly foods in Part Two of this book and a sample 4-day meal plan on page 164.

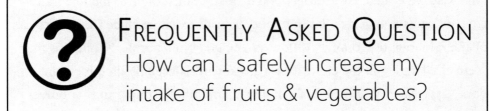

FREQUENTLY ASKED QUESTION
How can I safely increase my intake of fruits & vegetables?

Juices, smoothies, and purees are my favorite GP-friendly ways to increase fruit and veggie consumption and get more color into the diet.

Fresh Juices

Juicing removes almost all of the fiber from produce while retaining most of the nutrients and enzymes. Almost any fruit or vegetable can be juiced. Start with six ounces of juice diluted with up to an equal amount of water. Strain juice through a fine mesh strainer to remove pulp before drinking. Avoid high-FODMAP fruits and veggies like apples, pears, and beets unless you know that you are not sensitive.

Smoothies

Unlike juicing, blending does not remove the fiber in fruits and vegetables but it can make them easier to digest. Start with a small volume, no more than eight ounces, and experiment to determine which combinations of fruit, veggies, liquids, protein, and fat sources you tolerate best. For GP-friendly smoothie recipes, see pages 96-104.

Baby Food & Purees

Incorporating baby food into your diet can be a safe and convenient way to consume produce that you may not otherwise tolerate, such as berries and greens. Baby food is, after all, just pureed fruits and veggies. Try adding fruits to hot cereal or mixing vegetables into mashed potatoes. You can make your own "baby food" at home by simply cooking and pureeing your choice of fruits and veggies. See page 106.

One easy way to increase variety and diversify nutrition is to include more colorful fruits and vegetables in your diet. Aim to eat produce from all colors of the rainbow: red, orange, yellow, green, and blue/purple. While this may seem challenging in the context of a gastroparesis-friendly diet, it can be done, *especially* if you include fresh juices, smoothies, soups, and/or purees.

For examples of GP-friendly fruits and veggies in each color, see page 49.

Supplement with Nutrient-Rich Liquids and Soft Foods, as Necessary

For most people with mild to moderate symptoms, an all liquid diet is not necessary to manage gastroparesis. However, since liquids usually empty from the stomach more quickly than solids, alternating and/or supplementing liquid meals with solid meals may decrease symptoms, enhance nutrition, and help prevent unintentional weight loss.

You may be able to tolerate certain foods better in liquid form than in solid. For example, drinking raw carrot juice is less likely to provoke symptoms than eating raw carrots, just as drinking a green smoothie may be better tolerated than eating whole leafy greens.

When it comes to choosing liquids and soft foods, I recommend avoiding wheat, dairy, artificial sweeteners, and high-fructose corn syrup, especially while in a flare-up. (For more information on potentially gut-irritating foods, see page 33.)

Nutrient-rich liquids/soft foods include:

- Homemade bone broth

- Homemade gelatin
- Fruit, vegetable, and/or meat purees
- Mashed potatoes, sweet potatoes, or other root veggies
- Pureed soups
- Cream of buckwheat or cream of rice cereal
- Fruit/vegetable smoothies
- Fresh fruit/vegetable juice
- Meal replacement drinks (see notes below)

Meal Replacement Drinks

Most liquid meal-replacements contain a balance of carbohydrates, protein, and fat, as well as added vitamins and minerals. There are several to choose from, but not all are equally well-tolerated nor equally nourishing. I recommend Orgain (either Original or Vegan) over all other products currently on the market (I have no affiliation with the company).

For more information, visit the Book Resources page at www.EatingForGastroparesis.com.

Chew Thoroughly

Though we often overlook it, digestion begins in the mouth. Chewing not only prevents us from choking, it also mechanically breaks down food particles and allows them to mix with the enzymes in our saliva that help to digest carbohydrates and fat. The longer you chew your food, the easier the stomach's job becomes.

Chewing also signals the stomach to begin releasing gastric juices and ready itself for digestion. To best support the digestive process, eat slowly, chewing each bite until it's nearly the consistency of liquid. For nutrient-rich bever-

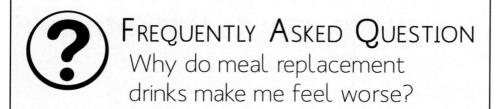

FREQUENTLY ASKED QUESTION
Why do meal replacement drinks make me feel worse?

Though meal replacement drinks, like Boost, Ensure, and Carnation Instant Breakfast, are frequently recommended for those with gastroparesis, some people will find that these products seem to worsen their digestive symptoms. There are several possible explanations.

Meal replacement drinks are formulated to contain fat, protein, carbohydrates, vitamins, and minerals. Because they are nutrient-dense, they empty more slowly than other liquids. The slower emptying time may account for an increase in symptoms.

Volume may also be a factor. Whereas most people with gastroparesis are conscious of their portion sizes when eating solid food, it's easy to consume a larger quantity of liquid in a short period of time. Make an effort to sip your beverages, drinking them slowly over time and holding each sip in your mouth for just a moment to begin digestion.

My opinion, though, is that the main problem with these products is their ingredients. They often contain high-fructose corn syrup, sugar alcohols, soy, and/or added fiber, all things that can exacerbate gastrointestinal symptoms.

I suggest trying Orgain, a newer product that does not contain any of the ingredients listed above. Orgain comes in two versions: Original, which is whey-protein based, and Vegan, which is plant-protein based. Many people find Orgain easier to tolerate (and tastier, too!).

ages, such as meal replacement drinks and smoothies, hold each sip in your mouth for just a moment before swallowing to allow the enzymes to begin working. This very simple act can make a significant difference, especially for those with compromised digestive function.

Eat Calmly and in a Relaxed Environment

How we eat can be just as important as *what* we eat when it comes to preventing and reducing symptoms associated with meal times. This is a result of what's called the Stress Response, a physiological process that occurs whenever our brain senses a threat.

When the Stress Response, also known as the "fight or flight" response, kicks in, the sympathetic nervous system takes over and hormones such as cortisol and adrenaline are released. Heart rate, blood pressure, and blood sugar increase. Blood flow is diverted away from the brain and digestive organs, going instead to the heart and the extremities. The release of gastric enzymes decreases significantly and the churning action of the stomach stops.

In a true emergency, this response enables us to fight or run for our lives. Unfortunately, the primitive area of the brain that triggers the Stress Response cannot differentiate between a true threat and an everyday stressor like an argument with your significant other -- or even an imagined threat, such as being worried that the food on your plate *may* give you a stomach ache.

Whatever the trigger, the reaction to stress, fear, worry, or anxiety is the same. The Stress Response kicks in and digestion essentially shuts down. You can see why this becomes a problem for those with gastroparesis when mealtime itself is hurried, tense, or otherwise stressful.

It's very important to make your eating environment and behaviors relaxed.

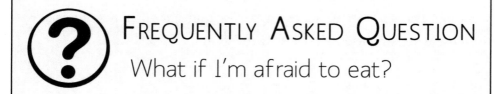

FREQUENTLY ASKED QUESTION
What if I'm afraid to eat?

It's not uncommon for those with gastroparesis to become fearful of straying from "safe" foods or even fearful of eating in general. If you're experiencing these feelings, it's important to address them as soon as possible.

By provoking the Stress Response, mealtime anxiety impairs digestion (separate from gastroparesis), often increasing symptoms. Experiencing symptoms may then heighten your fear of eating, creating a cycle that compromises both nutrition and symptom management.

It might help to remember that dietary modifications are a symptom-management tool for gastroparesis, not a treatment for gastroparesis. Eating something that doesn't agree with you will not affect your overall gastric emptying, nor will it make the condition more severe in the long-term.

You may also find it helpful to keep a food journal. This will allow you to see on paper what actually happens when you try new foods. You may be surprised how many foods you actually tolerate without added symptoms. See page 21.

If you find that you're unable to solve feelings of food-related anxiety on your own, consider working with a professional. To find a qualified counselor in your area, visit: http://therapists.psychologytoday.com.

Avoid eating while driving, while watching the news, or while having a heated discussion. Try not to rush through your meal or eat with people who make you feel self-conscious or defensive about the food on your plate.

It may be best to avoid eating if you are upset or otherwise stressed. Actively work to calm the body first, whether through deep breathing, journaling, going for a walk, meditating, practicing EFT (tapping), or simply removing yourself from a stressful situation. Then sit down and eat your meal.

Reduce or Eliminate Certain Foods

Aside from the general dietary guidelines about fat and fiber, there are certain foods that I believe warrant careful examination and experimentation, especially when symptoms are not well-controlled on a general nutrient-rich, GP-friendly diet.

Wheat/Gluten

Like many other nutrition professionals, my stance on gluten has changed dramatically in recent years. It is now my recommendation that those with gastroparesis eliminate all gluten-containing grains from their diet, at least initially. There are a number of reasons for this.

Gluten is a protein found in wheat, rye, and barley that often irritates the gut and may contribute to inflammation and additional food sensitivities. Grains that contain gluten are also high in fructans, a fermentable carbohydrate that can worsen digestive symptoms, especially for those with functional gut disorders. So whether it's the gluten or the FODMAPs, eliminating wheat, rye, and barley will often help to decrease digestive symptoms.

In addition, most of the gluten-containing foods in a GP-friendly diet are processed, refined foods that offer little if any nutritional value. From a nutritional standpoint, food products like white bread, pasta, cereal, cookies, crackers, and pretzels should not be consumed regularly. At best, they contribute no nutritional value. At worst they may exacerbate symptoms, impair the absorption of nutrients, and contribute to worsening gut health.

Dairy

My stance on dairy has also changed over the past several years. While I do believe that dairy can be part of a healthy, well-balanced diet, I've found that many people with gastroparesis benefit from removing it. Since dairy is so ubiquitous, both in the standard American diet and in the standard gastroparesis-friendly diet, you may not even realize that it's contributing to your symptoms until you stop consuming it for a period of time.

Similar to gluten, there are several explanations for the gastrointestinal symptoms associated with dairy products. Symptoms like nausea, bloating, gas, pain, and constipation may be the result of a sensitivity to the dairy protein, called casein, or an inability to absorb the dairy sugar, called lactose. Either way, removing dairy products from the diet for at least a couple of weeks will help you to evaluate whether they are adding to your distress.

In some cases, fermented dairy products, such as kefir and yogurt, may be better tolerated and provide healthy gut bacteria. Always choose organic dairy products to avoid antibiotics and hormones, and look for ones without added sugars, flavors, or colors.

Soy

Soy is difficult to digest, especially processed soy products like milk, ice cream, protein powders, and meat substitutes. Soy is also a common food sensitivity, as well as another source of fermentable carbohydrates (FODMAPs). All of this may lead to increased symptoms of nausea, pain, gas,

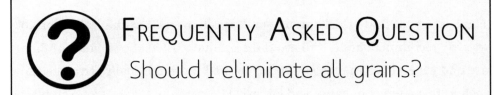

FREQUENTLY ASKED QUESTION
Should I eliminate all grains?

Paleo and Primal diets are becoming more popular and for good reason. When approached correctly, these diets promote a nutrient-rich whole foods diet focused on vegetables and fruits, high-quality fats, nuts, seeds, and moderate amounts of properly-raised animal protein.

These plans also eliminate all grains, due to the gut-irritating lechtins and phytase they contain. While I believe that eliminating grains *can* improve digestion, I don't think it's necessary or appropriate for everyone.

I do, however, strongly believe that the majority of GPers would benefit from eliminating all wheat and refined grain products. I also think it's important that all grains are prepared in a manner that supports optimal nutrition and digestion (page 146).

For those who wish to experiment with a grain-free diet, it's essential to make some gastroparesis-friendly modifications:

- Choose easier digested fats like coconut oil, red palm oil, and ghee over saturated fats like lard and tallow.
- Choose lean cuts of meat, ground meat, and slow-cooked meat.
- Eat more high-quality fish, an easily digested source of protein.
- Include plenty of GP-friendly carbs, such as roots, tubers, starchy vegetables, and tolerated fruits.
- Minimize grain-free baked goods, as they tend to be high in fat, fiber, and FODMAPs due to the use of coconut and almond flour.

and/or bloating.

There is a great deal of debate surrounding the overall health implications of soy. My recommendation is to avoid the products listed above, both for digestive and general health reasons, opting instead for traditionally fermented soy, such as miso, tempeh, natto, and tamari. These products are often well-tolerated by those who are not sensitive to soy in general.

Over 90% of the soy grown in the United States is genetically modified. The implications of this are unclear but concerning enough that I suggest sticking to certified organic products, which are free of GMOs, if you do choose to include soy in your diet.

Legumes

While most people with gastroparesis already know to avoid beans due to their high fiber content and propensity to increase gas, bloating, and abdominal pain, I think it's worth pointing out that peanuts are also legumes and may be difficult for some people to digest. If you don't do well with peanut butter, experiment with true nut butters or even seed butter. You may find that you tolerate those much better.

FODMAPs

FODMAPs are highly-fermentable carbohydrates that are often poorly digested and absorbed, particularly by those with functional gastrointestinal disorders. Because they're poorly absorbed, they provide fast food for our gut bacteria. For those of us with an imbalance of bacteria in our gut, bacteria growing in the wrong places (small intestinal bacterial overgrowth), or an increased sensitivity to sensations in the gut (visceral hypersensitivity), feeding those bacteria causes gas, bloating, pain, and bowel disturbances.

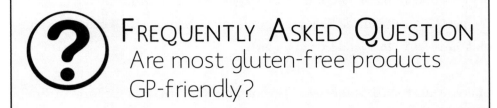

FREQUENTLY ASKED QUESTION
Are most gluten-free products GP-friendly?

It depends. In general I do not suggest replacing wheat-based snack foods, such as cookies, crackers, pretzels, and candy, with their gluten-free counterparts. These foods, though potentially less damaging without the gluten, are still for the most part empty, refined foods that fill your belly without nourishing your body. Additionally, there are some common ingredients in gluten-free processed foods that may provoke symptoms, including high-fiber gums and flours.

For the sake of convenience and sanity, however, it can be helpful to keep gluten-free staples like pasta and bread on hand. When choosing these products, look for the following:

- No more than 2-3 grams of fiber per serving, taking into account how many servings you plan to eat at one time.

- No bean flours, which can significantly increase fiber content, as well as the likelihood of subsequent bloating, gas, and pain.

- No chicory root, inulin, and FOS which are all sources of poorly-digested added fiber.

Keep in mind that brown rice flour, used in many gluten-free products, may increase constipation. Avoid frequent consumption if you struggle to have regular bowel movements.

Unfortunately some of the foods highest in FODMAPs are also the ones that many people think of as GP-friendly staples, including white bread, crackers, pasta, cereal, pancakes, applesauce, canned pears, canned peaches, skim milk, low-fat yogurt, and frozen yogurt.

Many meal replacement drinks also contain FODMAPs in the form of FOS, inulin, or chicory root. FODMAPs are often found in sports drinks and vitamin-infused waters in the form of high-fructose corn syrup and/or sugar alcohols. Most store-bought chicken, vegetable, and beef broths are high in FODMAPs due to ingredients like onion and garlic.

Temporarily eliminating high-FODMAP foods often helps to alleviate the symptoms mentioned above. While the diet has only been studied for IBS, I've found personally and in my coaching programs that it seems to be quite effective for many people with gastroparesis, as well. When a general nutrient-rich GP-friendly diet does not seem to alleviate symptoms of bloating, gas, and pain, a FODMAP elimination and reintroduction diet can be a helpful next step.

For more information, please visit the Book Resources page at www.EatingForGastroparesis.com.

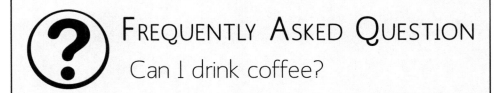

FREQUENTLY ASKED QUESTION
Can I drink coffee?

Coffee (both regular and decaf) contains tannins, which are irritating to the digestive tract. However, whether or not to completely eliminate it from your diet is a personal decision based on what makes you feel your best. Some people actually find that a moderate amount of coffee improves their symptoms, possibly due to it's ability to stimulate the lower gastrointestinal tract.

If you choose to drink coffee, please note that caffeine can take up to twelve hours to metabolize from the body. Avoid caffeinated beverages after mid-morning to support restful sleep.

Caffeine can also impact the adrenal glands, triggering a Stress Response of sorts, especially when consumed on an empty stomach. This may raise blood sugar, increase anxiety, and compromise weight management. If you choose to have a cup of coffee to start your day, drink it along with a well-balanced breakfast to minimize these effects.

Be mindful of what you add to your coffee. Avoid artificial sweeteners, which have both general health and specific digestive implications. Stick to regular sugar or pure stevia to sweeten your coffee. Avoid flavored creamers, as well, which typically contain trans fats, high fructose corn syrup, and other undesirable ingredients (see page 54). Opt instead for coconut milk, almond milk, or a splash of half-and-half if you tolerate dairy.

PART TWO:
SHOPPING & COOKING

Now that you're familiar with the basic guidelines of a health-promoting gastroparesis-friendly diet, it's time to think about what you're actually going to eat. On the following pages, you'll find a lengthy list of GP-friendly foods. My hope is that it will alleviate some of the overwhelm you may be feeling and illustrate just how many foods are still available for you to eat and enjoy -- despite the limitations of a gastroparesis-friendly diet.

This list is not conclusive and is not intended as a one-size fits all resource. There may be things on this list that *will not* work for you. On the other hand, there are likely to be things that are not on this list that *will* work for you. Don't be afraid to experiment as you become more familiar with the general dietary guidelines and your own personal tolerances.

Figuring out exactly what to buy, cook, and eat may seem time-consuming at first, but it does get easier and I urge you to vary your dietary choices as much as possible as you move forward. Keeping a wide variety of well-tolerated, GP-friendly options and recipes on hand will help to minimize the stress, boredom, and nutritional deficiencies that are often associated with a limited diet.

The Gastroparesis-Friendly Shopping List

While this list is designed to be a shopping list of sorts, you can also use it as a reference for choosing foods when eating in restaurants or at social gatherings. Where necessary, I've indicated how to prepare the foods in a gastroparesis-friendly manner.

Items marked with a pound sign (#) are foods with little nutrient value. These should not become dietary staples or take the place of more nutritious foods.

Items marked with an asterisk (*) are high-FODMAP based on the information available at the time this book was printed. Some of these foods may be tolerated in small quantities even while on a low-FODMAP diet. I highly suggest working with a knowledgeable nutrition professional if you are currently following a FODMAP elimination diet.

Items marked with a plus sign (+) are either higher in fiber or otherwise difficult for some people to digest due to common sensitivities and intolerances. Experiment with these foods to determine your tolerance.

Gastroparesis-Friendly Foods & Ingredients

Fat & Oils

Be cognizant of the amount of fat used. Each tablespoon of oil contains 14 grams of fat. Butter and ghee contain 11 grams per tablespoon.

- Butter +
- Coconut oil
- Ghee
- Olive oil
- Palm shortening
- Red palm oil

Seasonings & Spices

All spices are technically "gastroparesis-friendly" but you may find that there are some you do not tolerate, such as black and red pepper, chili powder, etc. If you have an autoimmune condition, you may need to avoid all seed- and nightshade- based spices such as anise, cumin, fennel, nutmeg, and paprika. The spices listed below are the ones I use most in my recipes and find to be generally well-tolerated by those with GP.

- Basil
- Cinnamon
- Ginger
- Oregano
- Rosemary
- Sage
- Sea salt
- Thyme
- Turmeric

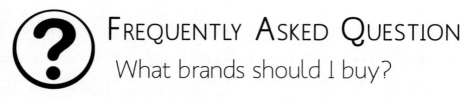

FREQUENTLY ASKED QUESTION
What brands should I buy?

If I think it's important to use a particular brand I have indicated that in the shopping list and the recipes that follow. Otherwise, I encourage you to choose those that best suit your budget and priorities.

For reference, here are the brands that I typically choose:
- Almond butter: Justin's Organic
- Bison/beef, sugar-free Canadian bacon: US Wellness Meats
- Buckwheat, millet: Eden Organic
- Coconut flakes (for homemade milk): Let's Do Organic
- Coconut oil, red palm oil: Nutiva or Tropical Traditions
- Chocolate Chips: Enjoy Life (Dairy/Soy Free)
- Gluten-free bread: Udi's White Sandwich Bread
- Gluten-free flours: Authentic Foods
- Gluten-free oats: Bob's Red Mill
- Gluten-free pancake mix: Arrowhead Mills
- Quinoa: TruRoots Sprouted Quinoa
- Olive oil: Kasandrino's
- Organic lean ground beef, pork, and turkey: Wegmans
- Palm shortening: Spectrum
- Salmon, cod: VitalChoice.com
- Salt: Pink Himalania Himalayan Pink Salt or Celtic Sea Salt
- Spices: Simply Organics
- Sunflower seed butter: Sunbutter Organic
- White rice: Lotus Foods Organic

Direct links to products can be found at www.EatingForGastroparesis.com.

Dairy/Nondairy Products

Look for products with the shortest ingredient lists. For ingredients to avoid, see page 54. You can also make your own nondairy milks at home. I've included several recipes in Part Three.

- Almond milk *
- Coconut milk, canned (light only)
- Coconut milk, refrigerated carton
- Flax milk
- Oat milk *
- Quinoa milk
- Rice milk

- Coconut milk kefir or yogurt
- Cow's milk kefir or yogurt, plain/unflavored +
- Parmesan cheese +

Protein

Most sources of lean protein are gastroparesis-friendly. Not all of them work well for everyone, though. Individual tolerances may depend on whether or not you have sufficient stomach acid, take medication for GERD, have any food sensitivities, and many other factors. Rather than assume that you don't tolerate animal protein, keep trying until you find the source(s) that are right for you at this time. In general, you'll want to avoid all fried meat, poultry, and seafood, opting instead for those that are baked, grilled, roasted, or slow cooked.

Meat/Poultry/Eggs
- Canadian bacon *US Wellness Meats recommended*
- Chicken breast, skinless
- Deli meat: ham, turkey breast, roast beef

? FREQUENTLY ASKED QUESTION
Should I buy Certified Organic?

While there is much debate as to whether organic food is more nutritious than its conventional counterpart, it is clear that buying Certified Organic food and food products reduces the amount of artificial ingredients and toxins in the diet. In the context of compromised digestion and an undernourished body, I think that's an important goal. Due to both cost and availability, it can be difficult to shop entirely organic. When prioritizing your food purchases, I recommend buying Certified Organic versions of the following whenever possible:

All Animal Products: Meat, Poultry, Milk & Eggs

What your meat eats, you eat. This goes for eggs and dairy products, too. Conventionally raised animals eat feed grown with conventional pesticides and fertilizers. It often contains genetically modified corn and soy, as well as animal by-products.

Conventionally raised animals are typically housed in overcrowded conditions that promote disease and are therefore routinely treated with antibiotics. Conventionally raised animals also frequently receive hormone injections to increase their size and/or production.

Organically raised animals, on the other hand, cannot receive antibiotics or growth hormones. Animals are fed grain, grass, and/or feed grown without chemical fertilizers or pesticides. No feed that includes GMOs or animal by-products is allowed. Overall, they are healthier animals and that means their milk, meat, and eggs are healthier, too.

Fruits & Vegetables

When we eat conventional produce, we consume pesticide and fertilizer residues and create more work for our digestion and detoxification systems. Eating organic produce reduces our toxic load, something that's good for the gut and for overall health. Organic produce can be expensive, so I recommend focusing on the Dirty Dozen.

This list is current as of 2014. For an updated list, please visit www.EWG.org.

The Dirty Dozen

These contain the most pesticide and chemical residue. Washing and peeling the produce will not remove it. Buy certified organic whenever possible.

1. Apple
2. Strawberries
3. Grapes
4. Celery
5. Peaches
6. Spinach
7. Sweet bell pepper
8. Nectarines (imported)
9. Cucumbers
10. Cherry tomatoes
11. Snap peas (imported)
12. Potatoes

The Clean Sixteen

These contain the lowest amount of chemical residue and/or are protected by a thick outer skin. Buy conventional to save money.

1. Avocados
2. Sweet corn
3. Pineapple
4. Cabbage
5. Sweet peas (frozen)
6. Onions
7. Asparagus
8. Mangoes
9. Papayas
10. Kiwi
11. Eggplant
12. Grapefruit
13. Cantaloupe
14. Cauliflower
15. Sweet potatoes
16. Mushrooms

- Eggs: whole
- Ground meat/poultry: beef, bison, pork, turkey (at least 90% lean)
- Hot dogs: chicken or turkey *Applegate Farms recommended*
- Liver: beef or chicken
- Sausage: chicken or turkey
- Turkey breast, skinless
- Turkey bacon *Applegate Farms recommended*
- Venison and other wild game

Fish/Seafood
- Cod
- Crab
- Haddock
- Halibut
- Lobster
- Orange Roughy
- Salmon, canned (packed in water)
- Salmon, fresh (wild-caught)
- Shrimp
- Tilapia
- Tuna fish, canned (packed in water)

Nut Butters & Substitutes

Two tablespoons per day is typically well-tolerated; choose smooth or creamy varieties only. Avoid products that contain hydrogenated or partially-hydrogenated oils. Also avoid low-fat varieties, which contain added oils and sugars.

- Almond butter
- Cashew butter *
- Macadamia nut butter
- Peanut butter +

- PB2: Powdered Peanut Butter ® +
- Pecan butter
- Pumpkin seed butter
- Sunflower seed butter
- Walnut butter

Fresh/Frozen Fruits

While most raw fruits are not GP-friendly, there are GP-friendly ways to consume them. I'm including those next to each fruit in parenthesis.

Red

- Grapes, red (juiced)
- Strawberries (juiced)
- Tomatoes (no skin or seeds; strained sauce; juice) +
- Watermelon (raw) *

Orange

- Cantaloupe (raw)
- Mangos (juiced, pureed) *
- Papaya (pureed, juiced, smoothies)
- Peaches (cooked/stewed, juiced, smoothies) *
- Squash: butternut (seeds removed; mashed, pureed) +

Yellow

- Pineapple (juiced, smoothies)
- Squash: summer (seeds removed; well-cooked)
- Squash: spaghetti (seeds removed; well-cooked) + *

Green

- Cucumber (juiced)
- Grapes, green (juiced)

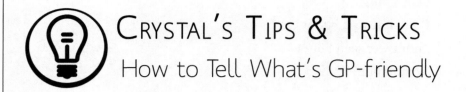

CRYSTAL'S TIPS & TRICKS
How to Tell What's GP-friendly

People often email me about foods, asking, "Is this GP-friendly?" While I can't always give a definitive answer, here's what I take into consideration -- and the things you can use yourself to decide whether various products are GP-friendly. Keep in mind that this is only a guide to help you determine what may and may not work for you. Careful experimentation will provide your best answer.

Serving Size

Always check the serving size of a product first, as the nutrition facts are based on one serving. For example, if you typically eat one cup of cereal and the serving size on the package is listed as one-half of a cup, you'll need to multiply all of the nutrition facts by two.

Fat

First, be sure that the product contains no trans fat. If it does, put it back. Otherwise, you'll want to evaluate the fat content based on how you plan to consume the food. If it's your entire meal and you only eat the amount in one serving size, then up to 10 grams of fat may be reasonable. On the other hand, if it will be a snack, only one part of your meal, or you tend to eat several servings at once, you'll want to look for a much lower fat content, maybe 3 grams per serving.

Fiber

The fiber content must be considered in a similar context as the fat content, although the window of tolerability tends to be smaller. It's unlikely, for example, that a product with 5 or more grams of fiber per serving would be considered GP-friendly. A general guideline is to choose products with less than four grams of fiber per serving, assuming you're only eating one serving. If you're going to eat multiple servings, one gram per serving may be a more appropriate limit.

Sugar

While sugar has traditionally been considered "GP-friendly" we now know that it can have significant impacts on the body, brain, and gut. I encourage you to reduce your sugar intake as much as possible, especially added and refined sugars.

Four grams of sugar is equal to about one teaspoon. To figure out how many teaspoons of sugar are in a product, divide the total grams of sugar by four. Don't forget to multiply by the number of servings you'll consume. This can be an eye-opening exercise, especially when it comes to sports drinks and sodas, which often have upwards of 10 teaspoons of sugar per bottle. Both the World Health Organization and the American Heart Association recommend consuming no more than 6 teaspoons of sugar per day.

Ingredients

Finally, check the ingredient panel, looking for ingredients that are not gastroparesis-friendly, such as whole nuts and seeds. See page 54 for additional ingredients you'll want to avoid.

Note that ingredients are always listed in order of amount used, from most to least. For example, if sugar is the first ingredient on a label, there is more sugar in that product than any other ingredient. This can be useful when determining whether or not a "healthy" product is actually healthy.

- Honeydew (raw)
- Zucchini (seeds removed; cooked)

Blue / Purple
- Blueberries (juiced)
- Grapes, black (juiced)

White
- Apples (applesauce, juice, stewed) +
- Bananas (raw, roasted, smoothies)
- Pears (cooked/stewed, juiced, roasted)

Fresh/Frozen Vegetables

While most raw vegetables are not GP-friendly, there are GP-friendly ways to consume them. I'm including those next to each vegetable in parenthesis.

Red
- Beets (juiced, roasted, pureed) *
- Roasted red peppers (skin and seeds removed; whole or pureed)

Orange
- Carrots (juiced, roasted, pureed, soups)
- Sweet potatoes (no skin; baked, mashed or pureed) +

Yellow
- Yellow carrots (juiced, roasted, pureed, soups)
- Roasted yellow peppers (skin and seeds removed; whole or pureed)

Green
- Leafy greens: all (juiced)
- Parsnips (roasted, pureed, soups) +

- Peas (well-cooked, pureed) +
- Spinach (juiced, smoothies, sautéed, soups, pureed)

Blue/Purple
- Purple carrots
- Purple potatoes

White
- Jersey White sweet potato (roasted, pureed, mashed, soups)
- Parsnips (roasted, pureed, soups)
- Turnips (roasted, pureed, soups) +
- White potatoes (no skin; baked, boiled, mashed, roasted, soups)

Non-perishables
- Applesauce *
- Baby food: assorted fruits and vegetables
- Canned pumpkin (solid pack; no more than 1/4 cup)
- Rao's Sensitive Formula Marinara Sauce (strain before using) +

Miscellaneous
- Almonds, raw (for homemade milk only) *
- Apple cider vinegar* *Braggs recommended*
- Chocolate chips (for baking) *Enjoy Life recommended*
- Cocoa powder (unsweetened) *
- Coconut flakes (unsweetened; for homemade milk only)
- Gelatin, unflavored *Great Lakes Kosher brand* **only**
- Maple syrup (not pancake syrup)
- Sugar (cane, raw if possible)

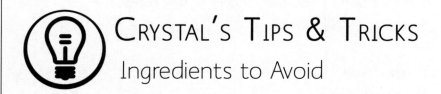

CRYSTAL'S TIPS & TRICKS
Ingredients to Avoid

By now you know to avoid non-GP-friendly ingredients like whole nuts, chia seeds, flax seeds, and potential bezoar contributors. There are other common ingredients, though, that can have a significant impact on digestion, nutrition, and overall health. I suggest avoiding the following whenever possible.

Carrageenan

Carrageenan is an ingredient used in many nondairy milks and meal replacement drinks to improve the texture. There is evidence that it is a gut irritant and promotes inflammation. I believe it's best to avoid regular consumption of carrageenan.

Inulin, chicory root, and FOS

Inulin, chicory root, and fructooligosaccharides (FOS) are indigestible carbohydrates, usually added to foods to increase the fiber content or sweetness. They're often found in yogurt, cereal, meal replacement shakes, protein bars, and probiotic supplements. The problem with these ingredients is two fold. Not only are they sources of added fiber, they are highly fermentable and may exacerbate bloating, gas, pain, and bowel problems, especially in those with functional gut disorders.

Artificial sweeteners

Artificial sweeteners, including Splenda (sucralose), aspartame (Equal), saccharin (Sweet 'n' Low), and acesulfame potassium (Sweet One), are used to sweeten everything from diet drinks to ice cream to jelly without adding calories. There is evidence, however, that these sweeteners contribute to hypoglycemia and sugar cravings, stimulate appetite, and may increase the risk of Type 2 Diabetes. Sucralose in particular has also been found to decrease beneficial gut bacteria.

Sugar alcohols

Sugar alcohols are artificial sweeteners that end in -ol. Examples are mannitol, sorbitol, and erythritol (found in Truvia and low-calorie vitamin waters). In addition to the problems with artificial sweeteners in general, sugar alcohols are highly fermentable and may exacerbate bloating, gas, pain, and diarrhea in those sensitive to FODMAPs.

High fructose corn syrup (HFCS)

While it's true that calorically there is no difference between HFCS and regular sugar, there is a significant difference in how these two ingredients are digested and absorbed, particularly for those with digestive issues. High fructose corn syrup is, as the name indicates, high in fructose. Fructose is commonly malabsorbed and may increase symptoms of bloating, gas, pain, and bowel irregularities.

Partially hydrogenated oils

Partially hydrogenated oils, found in cookies, crackers, protein bars, and many other products, are sources of trans fat. Trans fats are twice as hard for the body to break down as saturated fat. They decrease good cholesterol, increase bad cholesterol, and promote inflammation. Manufacturers can legally advertise a product as having zero grams of trans fat as long as there's less than .5 grams of trans fat per serving. No amount of trans fat belongs in the diet, so be sure to check for partially hydrogenated oils in the ingredient list.

Grains

Cold Cereals

- Puffed grains (rice, corn, etc.), without added sugar or ingredients
- *EnviroKidz* cereals #

Hot Cereals

- *Arrowhead Mills* Quinoa Rice & Shine
- Cream of Rice/Brown Rice Cream
- Cream of Buckwheat
- Oats, gluten-free (no more than 1/2 cup cooked per day) +
- Quinoa Flakes

Bread

- Gluten-free bread *Udi's White Sandwich Bread recommended*
- Spelt bread +

Flour/Starches

If you're going to do any gastroparesis-friendly baking, I recommend investing in the following pantry staples.

- Brown rice flour
- Millet flour
- Potato starch (not potato flour)
- Sorghum flour
- Tapioca flour
- Xanthan gum (to be used sparingly) +

Pasta

Choose gluten-free pastas with 2 grams of fiber or less per serving. Avoid pastas that contain bean flours.

- Buckwheat pasta
- Brown rice pasta
- Quinoa pasta

Whole Grains

- Buckwheat +
- Millet +
- Quinoa +
- White rice, any short or long grain variety

Protein Supplements/Meal Replacements

While meal replacements and protein supplements can play an important role in a GP-friendly diet, I encourage you to rely as much on whole food nutrition as possible. These products tend to be geared toward general ideas of what's "healthy" and that does not always correspond to what's ideal for gastroparesis management. Added fiber, whole nuts, chia seeds, flax seeds, and high-FODMAP ingredients, for example, may provoke symptoms even when found in a shake or protein powder. Read all ingredient lists and nutrition labels carefully before choosing supplements.

Unfortunately I do not know of a single meal replacement/protein supplement that I can universally suggest for GPers. Below are the products that I am most comfortable recommending for personal experimentation.

- MacroBars (Protein Purity *, Protein Pleasure +)
- Orgain: Original + or Vegan *
- Protein powder: Plant Fusion * or SunWarrior Classic Protein

Snacks

I encourage you to avoid packaged snack foods as much as possible, as they typically offer little nutrition. That said, these are my favorite GP-friendly options:

- Enjoy Life Sunbutter Crunch or Coco Loco Snack Bars *#
- EnviroKidz Crispy Rice Bars *#
- Inka Crops plantain chips (1 serving)

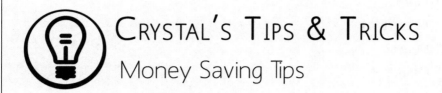

CRYSTAL'S TIPS & TRICKS
Money Saving Tips

A common tip for those who want to save money on groceries is, "shop around for the best prices." While this *is* a good tip, when you don't feel well and/or you've made self-care your first priority (good for you!), that's not always the best use of your time or energy. There are many other ways to reduce your food bill. Here are some of my GP-friendly favorites:

Use all of your scraps

Don't throw away the bones from your chicken or the peels from washed veggies: use them to make homemade stock! I store all bones and vegetable peels in the freezer in Ziplock bags until I have enough for a batch of stock. You'll find recipes for broth on pages 73-74.

Buy in bulk

Typically as the package size goes up, the price per unit goes down. Buy your grains, flours, oils, and meats in large family-sized packages. Be sure to properly store whatever you can't use immediately to preserve freshness. Flours, grains, and meats can all be stored in the freezer. Oils should be kept in a cool, dark place.

Sign up for email lists to receive coupons

While the majority of "clippable" grocery coupons are for nutrient-poor foods, manufacturers of pricey GP-friendly staples like coconut oil, nut butters, and spices often offer coupons for their products when you sign up for their mailing lists. Simply visit their websites and look for the link. *(This is a good project to reserve for a day when you're not feeling well and just want to lay in bed with your tablet or smart phone!)*

Focus on the Dirty Dozen

Organic produce is often significantly more expensive than conventional. Use the list on page 47 to get the most bang for your buck.

Subscribe & Save

Amazon.com's Subscribe & Save program offers discounts of 5-20% on thousands of grocery items. You choose how often you'd like to receive a shipment and you can cancel your shipments at anytime. Our family saves quite a bit by subscribing to many of our pantry staples, including nut/seed butters and coconut oil.

Plant a garden

Growing your own produce can drastically cut your grocery bill, especially if you tend to make a lot of juices, purees, or smoothies. Freeze your leftover harvest (nearly every fruit and vegetable can be frozen with minimal prep) and you'll save on food all year long. You'll also get the added health benefits of sunshine and mild physical activity as you take care of your garden.

Buy frozen

Depending on the time of year, one of my favorite ways to cut grocery costs is to buy frozen produce instead of fresh. This is especially economical if you make a lot of soups, purees, or smoothies using fruits and vegetables that aren't locally in season. You'll often be able to find coupons for frozen produce, as well. As a bonus, frozen fruits and veggies, which are frozen very soon after being picked, often contain more nutrients than their fresh counterparts that have traveled many miles and sat for days on store shelves.

PART THREE: GP-FRIENDLY RECIPES

In this section, I've included over 75 tasty recipes, everything from nutrient-rich liquids and soft foods to meals suitable for families and entertaining. My hope is that these recipes will enhance both the enjoyment *and* the nutritional quality of your diet, as well as help you achieve as much of a sense of "normalcy" as possible.

All of the recipes that follow are GP-friendly. In keeping with my recommendations, nearly all of the them are gluten-free, dairy-free, and soy-free. Of course, even with all of that taken into account, it does not mean that every recipe will be appropriate for you. Like everything else offered in this book, I encourage you to think of these recipes as a starting point for experimentation. You may find that you need to substitute certain ingredients or modify the recommended serving size based on your tolerances.

The number of servings listed on the recipes are GP-friendly servings, though typically large enough to feed others. If you will be making a recipe to feed only yourself, it's likely that you will get more servings out of it. If, on the other hand, you have family members with very hearty appetites, one serving may not be enough for them. In some cases, you'll notice a range of servings for this reason. The important part is that if you divide a recipe into the indicated number of servings, the amount of fat and fiber in each serving will be within general GP-friendly limits.

To the best of my knowledge, the majority of my recipes are low in FOD-MAPs with options provided for those who are not sensitive to FODMAPs and wish to broaden the variety in their diet. Recipes that are not low-FOD-MAP are indicated as such in the notes. If you are not sensitive to FOD-MAPs, feel free to use onions or shallots wherever I've called for green onion.

The low-FODMAP diet is relatively new and our knowledge about the FOD-MAP content of specific foods is constantly evolving. If you are following a low-FODMAP diet, it's best to work with a qualified professional to review which foods and recipes are and are not appropriate for you given the stage of the diet that you're in.

While all of my recipes are based on whole food nutrition with one of the goals being balanced blood sugar, they are not specifically designed for and may not always be appropriate for diabetics. If you are managing both gastro-paresis and diabetes, I encourage you to take this book to a nutrition professional specializing in diabetes and ask for their guidance in implementing the suggestions and recipes as part of your management plan.

You'll notice that nearly all of my recipes call for sea salt. Unless you're on a low-salt diet prescribed by your physician, don't be afraid of it! While sodium in canned and packaged foods is not health-promoting, sea salt added to home-cooked foods is a different story. In fact, lack of salt in the diet can contribute to low blood pressure, dizziness, and electrolyte imbalance.

You may also notice that none of my recipes include black pepper. That's because it's one ingredient that I neither like nor tolerate and therefore never include in my cooking. For those who can tolerate it, go ahead and add it anywhere you see fit.

Lastly, while you'll find over a dozen recipes for smoothies and juices in this section, I have also created a GP-Friendly Juicing & Blending eBook for those who would like more guidance and additional recipes. You can find that at http://bit.ly/gpjuicing.

With all of that out of the way... enjoy!

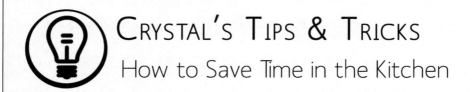

CRYSTAL'S TIPS & TRICKS
How to Save Time in the Kitchen

Use your slow cooker

A slow cooker is a great way to make GP-friendly meats and vegetables. The longer a meat is cooked, the easier it will be to eat and digest. I use my slow cooker so much that I bought a second one and now I often have both going at once! I use them not only to make stews but also to bake sweet potatoes, make broths, and cook whole chickens.

Plan your meals

Sit down once a week and plan out your family's meals. This eliminates the "what to cook" dilemma that's common around dinnertime. It also helps to prevent you from eating the same GP-friendly staples everyday simply because you don't know what else to make/eat.

Make one meal

When planning your meals, try to come up with several meals that you *and* the rest of your family can eat. Aim for at least the main dish to be GP-friendly. Even if you have to prepare additional side dishes for your family, it will be far less work than cooking two separate meals (or worse, skipping your meal altogether). There are many options for family-friendly meals in the recipes that follow.

Prep your staples

Prepare staples once a week to cut down on washing, chopping, soaking and cooking time. For example, we use a lot of ground meat and poultry, whole grains, and sweet potatoes, so I cook all of those in large batches at the beginning of the week and add them to recipes as needed.

If you plan to juice throughout the week, take one afternoon to wash and chop your fruits and veggies. They lose a bit of the nutrients but it saves a lot of time. Because it tends to help with consistency, I think this is a fair trade-off. (Alternately, you can make big batches of juice and freeze it in ice cubes to defrost throughout the week.)

Soak your grains

I describe the health benefits of soaking your grains on page 146, but it's a time-saver, too. Soaked grains cook up faster than unsoaked grains. You can cook a pot of soaked quinoa in about 15 minutes!

Use a pressure cooker

Pressure cookers are as easy to use as slow cookers and the newer ones come with a number of features that eliminate past safety concerns. Nutrient-rich bone broth in just one hour? Talk about a time-saver!

Stock your freezer

Having a freezer stocked with pre-portioned, homemade GP-friendly foods and ingredients makes incorporating more variety and nutrition easier. It can also alleviate the stress of cooking for family members, especially when you're not feeling well. So once a month I take a day to stock our freezer with soups, stews, and family-friendly heat and serve meals. I don't make enough for the whole month, of course, but once or twice a week, when there's nothing to eat and I don't want to cook, I pull something out and we have a healthy, home-cooked lunch or dinner.

For more tips on stocking your freezer, see page 116.

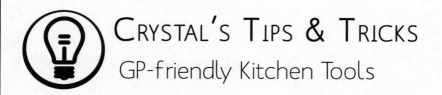

CRYSTAL'S TIPS & TRICKS
GP-friendly Kitchen Tools

Stocking your kitchen with the right tools will make cooking and preparing gastroparesis-friendly meals easier.

I recommend investing in the following (for the purpose indicated):
- Blender (for smoothies)
- Immersion blender or food processor (for soups and purees)
- Slow cooker (for broth, family meals, soups, etc.)
- Several 8 and 12 ounce freezer-safe containers (to freeze individual GP-friendly portions)
- Set of measuring cups (for experimenting with portion sizes)
- Steamer basket (for purees)
- Good knife and cutting board
- Vegetable peeler
- Cheesecloth/nut milk bag (for broth and nondairy milk)
- Digital thermometer (for cooking meat, poultry, and fish)
- Parchment paper (for baking without added fat)

These are optional but handy:
- Electric juicer (for fresh fruit and vegetable juices)
- Pressure cooker (for making broth, soups, grains, and more in a fraction of the time)
- Potato ricer or food mill (for potatoes and purees)
- Infantino pouch system (for purees)
- High-powered blender, such as Vitamix or Blendtec (can replace a food processor, immersion blender, and blender; for smoothies, soups, gluten-free flours, nut butters, etc.)

GP-FRIENDLY STAPLES

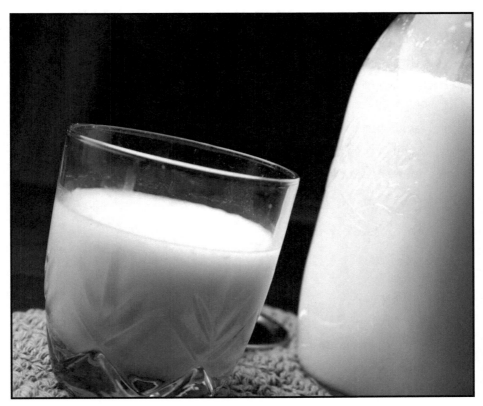

Coconut Milk, page 70

GINGER TEA

Ginger is a time-tested remedy for nausea and it has also been found to speed up gastric emptying, making this simple herbal tea ideal for symptom flare ups. If you aren't sensitive to fructose (a common FODMAP), use honey to sweeten up this spicy tea.

Ingredients

- 1-inch piece of fresh ginger
- 2 cups water
- honey and/or lemon, optional

Directions

1. Cut ginger into thin slices.
2. Bring water and ginger to a simmer in a small saucepan.
3. Simmer for 15–20 minutes. (For extra-strength ginger tea, simmer for up to 1 hour, until liquid is reduced by half.)
4. Remove from heat and strain out ginger slices.

GPNB (GPer's Nut Butter)

Nut butter is a nutrient-rich, satisfying source of GP-friendly fat. While most GPers tolerate at least one or two tablespoons per day, sometimes it's nice to have a little more wiggle room. Enter GPNB! The GPer's Nut Butter: all of the flavor, half the fat...

Ingredients

- 3/4 cup creamy nut or seed butter (peanut butter, almond butter, sunflower seed butter, etc.)
- 3/4 cup almond, light coconut, or quinoa milk
- 1 Tbsp pure maple syrup
- 1/4 tsp ground cinnamon, optional

Directions

1. Add milk, nut butter, maple syrup, and cinnamon (if desired) to a blender in that order.
2. Blend until smooth.
3. Store in the refrigerator in a tightly sealed container.

Notes

Use on toast, pancakes, waffles, hot cereal, cooked grains, and/or in smoothies. One two-tablespoon serving will contain approximately 8-10 grams of fat depending on your choice of milk and nut/seed butter.

COCONUT MILK

While coconut itself is high in fat, the more water you add to this milk, the thinner it will be and the less fat each cup will contain. I recommend starting with four cups of water and experimenting with more or less according to your tolerances and preference.

Ingredients

- 2 cups unsweetened coconut
- 4 to 6 cups of water, divided

Directions

1. Soak coconut flakes in 2 cups of water for 2-3 hours.
2. Pour coconut flakes and soaking water into your blender.
3. Add 2-4 more cups of water.
4. Blend 1-2 minutes, or until smooth.
5. Strain the mixture through cheesecloth or a nut milk bag.
6. Refrigerate and enjoy!

Notes

Coconut milk initially tested as high-FODMAP but recent testing has shown that it's actually low in FODMAPs. Some of the additives found in store bought coconut milks are not, though. Making it at home allows you to control both fat content and ingredients.

ALMOND MILK

Most recipes for almond milk call for one cup of almonds to four cups of water. The fat content in that ratio is often too high for GPers. I suggest starting with 6 cups of water and adjusting according to your tolerance. **Almond milk is not low-FODMAP.**

Ingredients

- 1 cup of almonds
- 10 cups of water, divided
- pinch of sea salt
- 1 tsp vanilla extract, optional
- maple syrup or honey to sweeten to taste, optional

Directions

1. Put almonds in a bowl and add about 4 cups of water. Place in the refrigerator and soak 8-12 hours.
2. Drain and rinse almonds.
3. Place almonds in a high-powered blender with 2 cups of water and blend until smooth, about 2 minutes.
4. Add 4 more cups of water and blend 1 more minute.
5. Strain through cheesecloth or a nut milk bag.
6. Stir in salt, sweetener, and/or extract, if desired.
7. Store the milk in the refrigerator for 4-5 days.

QUINOA MILK

Quinoa is rich in manganese, tryptophan, phosphorus, folate, and magnesium. Making milk out of the cooked grain removes the fiber while retaining many of the nutrients. The flavor is distinctive. I use it primarily in savory recipes or smoothies.

Ingredients

- 2 cups cooked quinoa
- 6 cups of water, divided
- 1 Tbsp maple syrup
- 1 tsp vanilla extract

Directions

1. Place the cooked quinoa and 2 more cups of water into a blender. Blend until smooth, about a minute.
2. Add the remaining 4 cups of water while blending, until it reaches desired consistency.
3. Add maple syrup and vanilla extract, if desired.
4. Strain the milk through a nut milk bag or piece of cheesecloth.
5. Store the milk in the refrigerator for 4-5 days.

VEGETABLE BROTH

Most vegetable broths contain onions and garlic, making them high in FODMAPs, and tomatoes, making them too acidic for many sensitive stomachs. This recipe avoids all of the above but is still flavor and nutrient-rich.

Ingredients

- 8 cups water
- 2 bay leaves
- 4 carrots
- 1 medium sweet potato
- 1/2 cup fresh parsley
- 1 stalk celery with leaves
- 1/2 cup chopped green onions (green part only)
- 2-inch piece of ginger, peeled
- 2 tsp sea salt

Directions

1. Wash and chop all vegetables. There is no need to peel clean organic vegetables.
2. Add all ingredients to a large stockpot.
3. Bring to a boil then reduce heat and simmer for 1 to 2 hours. Alternatively, add all ingredients to a slow cooker and cook on high for 4-6 hours.
4. Allow to cool.
5. Strain through a fine mesh strainer.
6. Store in the refrigerator for 4-5 days or freeze for later use.

HOMEMADE CHICKEN BROTH

Unlike store-bought broth, homemade chicken broth is incredibly nourishing, especially for those with digestive issues. The gelatin helps to heal the gut and facilitate digestion of other food, and the easily absorbed minerals help to strengthen the entire body.

Ingredients

- chicken carcass or 1 to 2 lbs of bones
- 10 cups water
- 2 Tbsp apple cider vinegar
- 4 carrots, peeled and chopped
- 10 chives, washed
- 2 bay leaves
- 2 tsp sea salt
- 1 tsp thyme
- 1/4 cup fresh parsley
- 2-inch piece of ginger, peeled, optional

Directions

1. Put bones in a large stockpot. Add water and vinegar.
2. Cover and let it sit for 30 minutes.
3. Bring to a gentle boil and skim off the "scum" (foam) that comes to the top.
4. Lower the heat and let the broth simmer 6-24 hours (the longer, the better!).
5. With four hours left to cook, add vegetables, herbs, and salt.
6. Allow finished broth to cool then strain through cheesecloth.
7. Store overnight in the refrigerator. Skim the solidified fat off the top and then refrigerate or freeze the finished broth.

SLOW COOKER BEEF BROTH

Beef broth tends to be fattier than chicken broth. You may find that drinking beef broth by itself exacerbates your symptoms for this reason, especially if you do not have a gallbladder. Using the broth in soups is often well-tolerated and very nourishing.

Ingredients

- 3 lbs beef bones
- water
- 4 carrots, peeled and chopped
- 2 Tbsp apple cider vinegar
- 2 bay leaves
- 2 tsp sea salt

Directions

1. Preheat oven to 450°F.
2. Arrange bones on a rimmed baking sheet and roast for 20-30 minutes, until browned.
3. Place roasted bones, carrots, vinegar, and seasonings in the slow cooker.
4. Fill slow cooker to the top with water.
5. Cook on low for 12 hours.
6. Strain broth through cheesecloth or a nut milk bag.
7. Chill broth in the refrigerator over night. Skim the solidified fat off the surface and then store in the refrigerator or freezer.

MULTI-TASKER CHICKEN

This is a time-saving recipe. Throw a whole chicken in the slow cooker, walk away, and in six hours you've got several cups of cooked chicken, plus a jump start on a 24-hour bone broth.

Ingredients

- whole chicken
- water

Directions

1. Put whole chicken in slow cooker. Cover with water.
2. Cook on low for six hours.
3. Remove chicken from slow cooker. Allow to cool.
4. Remove meat from the bones. Discard skin.
5. To make broth, place bones back in the slow cooker, adding more water if necessary. Cook on low for 12-18 more hours.

Notes

Use cooked chicken for GP-friendly soups and/or to prepare quick meals for your family throughout the week, such as stir fry, chicken fried rice, chicken salad, or fajitas.

BLUEBERRY GEL-O

Jello is junk food, full of sugar, artificial chemicals, and colors. Good quality gelatin from properly raised animals, however, has many health benefits and is especially healing for the digestive tract. When you're not feeling well or you simply need a nourishing treat, give this homemade Gel-O a try.

Ingredients

- 1-1/2 cups cold water
- 5 Tbsp 100% organic blueberry juice concentrate (or any flavor you like)
- 2 Tbsp Great Lakes Unflavored Kosher Beef Gelatin
- 1-1/2 cups hot water (not boiling)
- stevia or natural sweetener, to taste

Directions

1. Combine the cold water with the blueberry concentrate in a medium sized bowl.
2. Slowly add the gelatin, a little at a time, whisking constantly. (Don't be concerned about the smell of the gelatin. It will disappear after the Gel-O chills.)
3. Continue whisking for about a minute, until gelatin is dissolved.
4. Carefully stir in hot water.
5. Add stevia to taste, if desired.
6. Cover the bowl and chill in the refrigerator for at least 6 hours before serving.

ELECTROLYTE DRINK

This homemade "sports drink" contains all of the essential ingredients for hydration (water, salt, and sugar) without the artificial colors, flavors, and sweeteners of store-bought varieties. Coconut water and cucumber juice are also naturally rich in electrolytes. You can omit the lime juice if you do not tolerate citrus.

Ingredients

- 3-1/2 cups water
- 1/2 cup coconut water or cucumber juice (about 1 cucumber)
- 1/4 tsp Himalayan Pink Salt or Celtic Gray Salt
- 1 to 2 Tbsp maple syrup or honey, to taste
- juice of 1/2 lime, optional
- 2 tsp NaturalCalm plus Calcium, optional

Directions

1. Heat one cup of water over low heat. Add salt and sweetener, stirring until combined.
2. Add remaining water and coconut water/juice. *(Note that coconut water is FODMAP friendly in servings less than 1/3 cup.)*
3. Stir in optional ingredients, if desired.
4. Refrigerate.

BREAKFAST

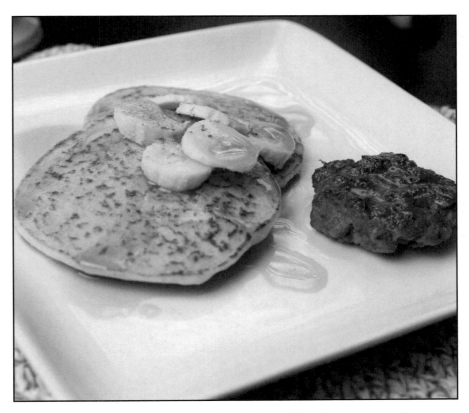

Quick & Easy Pancakes, page 92 and Baked Breakfast Sausage, page 83

BANANA PANCAKE FOR ONE

This one-serving pancake offers a good balance of protein, carbohydrates, and healthy fat to start your day. If you don't have oat flour, process whole gluten-free oats in a Vitamix or food processor until flour consistency.

Ingredients

- 1/4 cup gluten-free oat flour
- 1/2 tsp baking powder
- 1 medium ripe banana
- 1 egg, lightly beaten
- 1/2 tsp vanilla extract
- 1 to 2 Tbsp GPNB (see page 69)

Directions

1. In a small bowl, combine flour and baking powder.
2. Mash banana in a separate bowl.
3. Add egg and vanilla to the bananas. Stir until combined.
4. Stir the banana mixture into the dry ingredients just until moistened. Batter will be thick.
5. Pour batter onto a hot ceramic-coated nonstick skillet.
6. Cook until bubbles form on the surface, then flip and cook until golden brown.
7. Spread with GPNB.

Spelt Carrot Muffins

Spelt is an ancient form of wheat. It is not gluten-free but it does contain 5,000 times less gluten than modern wheat and may be well-tolerated by those with non-Celiac gluten sensitivity or FODMAP issues. Pair with protein and a little fat for breakfast.

Ingredients

- 2 cups shredded carrots
- 1 small banana, very ripe
- 1/2 cup pure maple syrup
- 1/4 cup melted coconut oil
- 1 egg or 1/4 cup applesauce
- half an orange, juiced

- 1-1/2 cups sprouted spelt flour *(recommended: Shiloh Farms)*
- 1/2 tsp baking soda
- 1/2 tsp baking powder
- 1-1/2 tsp cinnamon
- 1/2 tsp ginger

Directions

1. Preheat oven to 350°F. Fill a muffin tin with liners.
2. In a high-powered blender or food processor, combine first 6 ingredients. Puree until completely smooth.
3. In a large mixing bowl, combine all dry ingredients.
4. Pour wet ingredients into dry ingredients and stir just until moistened and combined.
5. Fill each muffin liner with about 1/3 cup of batter.
6. Bake for 18 minutes.
7. Cool on a wire rack.

PUMPKIN SPICE QUINOA & RICE

Between the pumpkin, cinnamon, and maple syrup, this nourishing breakfast tastes like Autumn in a bowl! I like the rice/quinoa blend because it has a bit more protein but cream of rice can be substituted. You may need an additional 1/4 cup of liquid.

Ingredients

- 1/4 cup uncooked Arrowhead Mills Quinoa Rice & Shine
- 1/2 cup water
- 1/4 cup light coconut milk
- 1/4 cup pumpkin puree
- 1/2 tsp cinnamon
- pinch of sea salt
- pinch of ginger
- 1 Tbsp almond butter
- 2 tsp maple syrup, optional

Directions

1. Combine millet, water, pumpkin, and spices in a sauce pan.
2. Bring to a boil over high heat. Cover, reduce heat, and simmer for 25-30 minutes.
3. Add more liquid depending on desired consistency.
4. Stir in maple syrup and serve.

BAKED BREAKFAST SAUSAGE

I hadn't had breakfast sausage in nearly a decade before I came up with the idea to make my own with lean meat and FODMAP-friendly spices. It's now a breakfast staple in our house and I'm happy to have it back! Adjust the seasonings to your tastes.

Ingredients

- 1 lb lean ground meat (turkey, chicken, beef, pork)
- 1 Tbsp maple syrup, optional
- 1 tsp sea salt
- 3/4 tsp ground sage
- 3/4 tsp dried thyme
- 1/4 tsp cinnamon

Directions

1. Preheat oven to 400°F. Line a rimmed baking sheet with aluminium foil for easy clean up.
2. Mix all ingredients by hand in a bowl.
3. Form into 8 small patties. Place on baking sheet.
4. Cook for 10 minutes. Flip patties and rotate pan.
5. Bake 10 more minutes or until the internal temperature reaches 165°F.

EASY BAKED EGGS

Eggs are a well-tolerated source of protein for many people with gastroparesis. Don't be afraid of the yolks – a whole egg, including the yolk, has less than 5 grams of fat and is packed with choline, B vitamins, and other nutrients not found in the white.

Ingredients

- 2 tsp butter or coconut oil
- 4 large eggs
- 1 tsp sea salt
- 4 tsp nondairy milk

Directions

1. Preheat oven to 350°F.
2. Coat 4 (6-ounce) ramekins with 1/2 tsp butter or oil.
3. Break 1 egg into each prepared ramekin.
4. Sprinkle eggs evenly with salt. Pour 1 teaspoon of milk over each egg.
5. Place ramekins in a 13 x 9-inch baking dish; add about 1 inch of hot water to pan.
6. Bake for 25 minutes or until eggs are set.

SPINACH & EGG CASSEROLE

Most egg casseroles call for fatty meats and heavy cream. This one is much lighter and healthier, but still tasty. If you tolerate dairy, definitely include the layer of Parmesan cheese on top. It's low-fat, low-FODMAP, and delicious!

Ingredients

- 8 whole eggs
- 1-3/4 cup almond or rice milk
- 2 cups cooked millet
- 1 cup baby spinach, finely chopped
- 1 tsp thyme
- 1/2 tsp salt
- 1/2 cup shredded Parmesan cheese, optional to taste

Directions

1. Preheat oven to 350°F.
2. Rub a 13 x 9-inch casserole dish with oil.
3. Whisk together eggs and milk until combined.
4. Stir in millet, spinach, and seasonings.
5. Pour into prepared pan.
6. Bake for 40-50 minutes, until eggs are set and slightly puffy.

Maple Sausage Hash

My husband always said he didn't like sweet potatoes -- until I made him this one-skillet breakfast! It's a well-balanced GP-friendly meal with healthy sources of fat, protein, and carbohydrates. I often drink my Daily Green Juice with it. (Page 94)

Ingredients

- 1 lb lean ground pork
- 1 Tbsp coconut oil
- 1 tsp sea salt, to taste
- 1/2 tsp sage
- 1/2 tsp thyme
- 1/2 tsp cinnamon

- 2 medium baked sweet potatoes, peeled and diced
- 1 Tbsp maple syrup

Directions

1. Melt coconut oil in a skillet over medium heat.
2. Add the pork to the skillet. Sprinkle with thyme and sage. Cook until no pink remains. Push to one side of the skillet.
3. Add the diced sweet potatoes to the other side of the skillet. Sprinkle with cinnamon.
4. Cook until the sweet potatoes start to brown, stirring occasionally, about 3-5 minutes. Drizzle with maple syrup.
5. Carefully mix the pork and the sweet potatoes together and serve.

TURKEY & CARROT HASH

Not to be confused with it's fattier counterpart, Canadian bacon is a low-fat, high-protein GP-friendly breakfast meat. It's optional but recommended in this dish! If you skip the bacon, simply start with step 3, adding 1-2 teaspoons coconut oil to the skillet.

Ingredients

- 1 tsp coconut oil
- 2 slices Canadian bacon, optional
- 1 lb ground turkey breast
- 4 carrots
- 1 tsp sea salt
- 1/2 tsp thyme

Directions

1. Heat oil in a skillet over medium heat.
2. Add bacon and cook until slightly brown on both sides. Set aside.
3. In the same skillet, cook turkey, thyme, and salt over medium heat until brown.
4. While the turkey is cooking, peel and shred the carrots.
5. Add shredded carrots to the skillet. Cover and reduce heat to low.
6. Cook for 5-7 minutes, until the carrots are softened.
7. Meanwhile chop the cooked bacon into small pieces.
8. Add bacon to skillet. Stir to combine.

Mix 'n' Match Hot Cereal

So many combinations! Experiment to find your favorite. Cooking times and amounts vary for each type of cereal, so prepare according to the directions on the package. Prepared individual portions can be frozen in storage containers for a quick and easy meal.

Choose a Cereal

- Cream of Rice/Brown Rice Cream – gluten-free; low in fiber
- Cream of Buckwheat - gluten-free; low in fiber
- Quinoa Flakes - gluten-free; higher protein; 2.6g fiber
- Arrowhead Mills Quinoa Rice & Shine - gluten-free; 2g fiber

Choose a Liquid

- water
- milk (almond, rice, or coconut)
- broth (chicken, beef, or vegetable)

Choose Add-Ins

- 1/4 to 1/2 cup homemade fruit puree or "baby food"
- ½ banana, mashed up
- ¼ cup canned pumpkin
- 1 Tbsp smooth peanut, almond, pecan, or sunflower seed butter
- 1 to 2 tsp coconut oil
- 1 scoop of protein powder
- 1 Tbsp Great Lakes Unflavored Kosher Collagen
- 1 Tbsp maple syrup
- cinnamon, ginger, or pumpkin pie spice, to taste

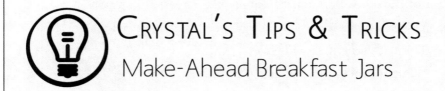

CRYSTAL'S TIPS & TRICKS
Make-Ahead Breakfast Jars

I started making these Breakfast Jars when my daughter was a new-born. One hour of cooking and jar prep yields a full week's worth of ready-to-go nutrient-rich breakfasts.

To prepare seven jars, you'll need 5-8 cups of cooked hot cereal. I recommend choosing two different kinds and alternating from week to week. Choose two or three "Add In" combinations, as well.

Then it's as easy as layering the ingredients in the jars. I like to start with the fruit, then layer nut/seed butters and/or coconut oil, followed by seasonings, and finally the cereal. Cover and refrigerate the layered jars until ready to use.

To reheat, either dump the contents into a pan and warm over medium-low heat or remove the lid and pop the jar in the microwave for about 60 seconds. Stir well and heat for an additional 30 seconds, if necessary.

Choose 8- or 12-ounce mason jars depending on your meal size tolerance (1 cup versus 1-1/2 cups). If you tolerate slightly larger meals but plan to add a protein source on the side, such as Baked Breakfast Sausage, 8-ounce jars are probably sufficient.

You'll find a few of my favorite Breakfast Jar combinations on the next page.

Peanut Butter & Banana Jar (approx. 8-9g fat; 3-3.5g fiber)

In an 8- or 12-ounce jar:

- 3/4 to 1 cup Quinoa Flakes
- 1/2 medium banana, mashed or pureed
- 1 Tbsp peanut butter

Blueberry Almond Jar (approx. 9.5g fat; 3.5-4g fiber)

In an 8- or 12-ounce jar:

- 3/4 to 1 cup Quinoa Rice 'n' Shine
- 1/4 cup blueberry puree ("baby food")
- 1 Tbsp almond butter
- pinch of sea salt

Nut-Free Pumpkin Jar (approx. 9g fat; 4g fiber)

In an 8-ounce jar:

- 3/4 cup cooked Brown Rice Cream
- 1/4 cup pumpkin
- 1 Tbsp Great Lakes Kosher Collagen
- 2 tsp maple syrup
- 2 tsp coconut oil
- 1/4 tsp cinnamon

Sweet Potato Pie Jar (approx. 9g fat; 4g fiber)

In an 8-ounce jar:

- 3/4 cup Cream of Buckwheat
- 1/4 cup mashed sweet potato
- 1 Tbsp walnut butter
- 2 tsp maple syrup, optional
- 1/4 tsp cinnamon
- pinch of sea salt

EASY GLUTEN-FREE WAFFLES

You can also make these as pancakes, cooking 2-3 minutes per side. I prefer letting the waffle iron do the work, though! For a well-balanced meal, be sure to include protein and a little healthy fat. A serving of Baked Breakfast Sausage (page 83) would work.

Ingredients

- 1 cup brown rice flour
- 1/4 cup millet flour
- 1/2 cup potato starch
- 1-1/2 Tbsp sugar
- 2 tsp baking powder
- 1/2 tsp sea salt

- 1 cup water
- 1/4 cup fruit puree (applesauce, pumpkin, banana, etc.)
- 2 Tbsp coconut oil, melted

Directions

1. Combine dry ingredients in a medium bowl.
2. Combine wet ingredients in a separate bowl.
3. Pour wet mixture into dry mixture, stirring to combine.
4. Grease waffle maker according to directions. (Non-stick models typically do not need to be oiled.)
5. Pour batter into waffle iron, using about 1/4 cup per waffle.
6. Cook according to waffle iron directions.
7. Serve with maple syrup or GPNB (page 69).

QUICK & EASY PANCAKES

I don't recommend pancakes everyday but once in a while, they're a wonderful treat!
I recently made these for a house full of guests and nobody believed that they were
gluten-free, vegan, and low-fat! Add a low-sugar protein source to complete your meal.

Ingredients

- 2 cups Arrowhead Mills Gluten-Free Pancake Mix
- 1 cup water
- 1/2 cup applesauce or other fruit puree
- 1 Tbsp coconut oil, melted
- 1 tsp vanilla extract

Directions

1. Heat a skillet over medium heat. Very lightly grease with palm shortening.
2. Mix all ingredients in a large bowl until combined. Do not over mix.
3. Scoop 1/4 of batter onto skillet for each pancake. Cook for 2-3 minutes or until bubbles form on the surface. Flip and cook for two more minutes or until cooked through.
4. Serve warm with GPNB or maple syrup.
5. Freeze any leftovers in freezer safe Ziplock bags with parchment paper between each pancake. Reheat in the toaster.

JUICES, SMOOTHIES & PUREES

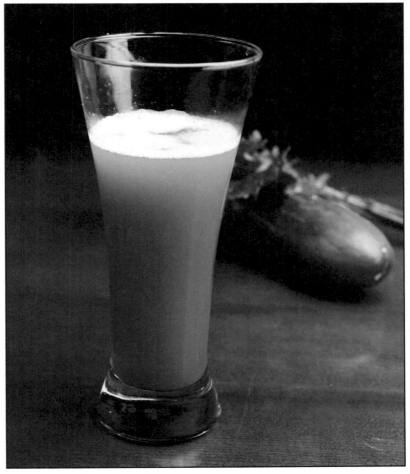

Daily Green Juice, page 94

DAILY GREEN JUICE

After quite a bit of experimentation, this has become my near-daily green juice. Pineapple contains natural digestive enzymes, but if you don't like or can't tolerate it, substitute red or green grapes instead.

Ingredients

- 1 cucumber, peeled
- 2 cups baby leafy greens (spinach, kale, chard, etc.)
- 1/2 cup pineapple chunks

Directions

1. Feed ingredients through an electric juicer in the order listed.
2. Strain juice through a fine-mesh strainer.
3. Dilute with water, if necessary.
4. Store leftover juice in the refrigerator in a tightly sealed container for up to 12 hours.

CARROT-GINGER JUICE

Ginger has anti-nausea properties and has been found to speed up gastric emptying when consumed regularly. It adds a slightly spicy flavor to this bright orange juice.

Ingredients

- 2 large carrots, peeled and chopped
- 1/2 cup green grapes, washed
- 1/2-inch piece of gingerroot, peeled

Directions

1. Feed all ingredients through the juicer.
2. Strain juice through a fine mesh strainer.
3. Dilute with 4 to 6 ounces of water, if necessary.

BERRY GOOD JUICE

Though berries aren't typically considered GP-friendly, their juice certainly is. Juicing removes the seeds and the fiber from the berries while preserving most of the enzymes and antioxidants. This is a great way to add more red and blue to your diet!

Ingredients

- 1 cup strawberries, washed and trimmed
- 1 cup blueberries, washed

Directions

1. Feed berries through the juicer.
2. Strain through a fine mesh strainer.
3. Dilute with 4 to 6 ounces of water, if necessary.

GRAPES & GREENS

The grapes really mellow the flavor of the kale in this simple but nutrient-rich juice. You can use any color grapes but red grapes contain the brain-boosting antioxidant resveratrol.

Ingredients

- 1 cup red grapes, washed
- 1 cup baby kale greens, washed

Directions

1. Feed ingredients through the juicer in the order listed.
2. Strain through a fine mesh strainer.
3. Dilute with 4 to 6 ounces of water, if necessary.

BASIC SMOOTHIE FORMULA

This isn't a recipe so much as a method. Smoothies are a convenient, often well-tolerated option for mini-meals and snacks. Mix and match according to your preferences and tolerances to find the combination that works best for you.

Ingredients

- 1 cup liquid (water, juice, non-dairy milk)
- 1 cup of fruit
- 1 handful of baby greens, optional

Add-Ins

- 1 to 2 Tbsp nut or seed butter
- 1 scoop protein powder
- 1 Tbsp Great Lakes Kosher Collagen
- 1 to 2 tsp coconut oil

Directions

1. Place ingredients in blender, starting with the liquid.
2. Blend until smooth.

Go-To Green Smoothie

This is an easy way to eat more greens. If you find that raw spinach exacerbates your symptoms, you can steam or sauté it first and cool completely before blending. The gelatin supplement is optional but so nourishing for digestion... include it if you can!

Ingredients

- 6 to 8 oz almond or light coconut milk
- 1 ripe banana, sliced and frozen
- 1 cup baby spinach
- 1 Tbsp Great Lakes Kosher Collagen, optional
- 1 Tbsp nut or seed butter, optional

Directions

1. Combine all ingredients in a blender.
2. Process until smooth.
3. Drink immediately.

RAINBOW SMOOTHIE

Though this recipe requires both a juicer and a good blender, it's worth the effort and clean up... it covers every color of the GP-friendly rainbow, after all!

Ingredients

- 2 carrots
- 1/2 cup seedless purple grapes
- 6 strawberries
- 1/2 medium ripe banana, frozen
- large handful of organic spinach leaves (about 1 cup)
- 2-4 oz water

Directions

1. Wash all produce. Peel the carrots and trim the tops off the strawberries.
2. Feed grapes, strawberries, and carrots through an electric juicer.
3. Strain juice to remove any remaining pulp.
4. In a blender, combine juice, banana, spinach, and 2 ounces of water.
5. Blend until well combined, adding more water as necessary.
6. Sip slowly and enjoy!

BANANA COLADA

This tastes like a frosty treat but there's no added sugar. I like it for a late afternoon snack. If you choose to drink it for breakfast, be sure to add the protein! I particularly like the flavor of Plant Fusion in this one, but use any protein powder you tolerate.

Ingredients

- 6 oz homemade coconut milk
- 1 banana, sliced and frozen
- 1/4 tsp vanilla extract
- 1 scoop vanilla Plant Fusion protein powder, optional

Directions

1. Combine all ingredients, in the order listed, in a blender.
2. Process until smooth.
3. Serve immediately.

PINA COLADA SMOOTHIE

I don't drink alcohol but I can never resist a virgin Pina Colada when I'm on vacation. Love the flavor! If you find even pureed pineapple too fibrous, you can omit it and still retain the flavor by replacing the water with pineapple juice and using 1 whole banana.

Ingredients

- 4 oz light coconut milk
- 2 to 4 oz water
- 1/2 banana, frozen
- 1/2 cup of diced pineapple, frozen
- 1 scoop vanilla protein powder, optional

Directions

1. Add ingredients to the blender in the order listed.
2. Blend until smooth, adding more liquid as necessary.

BANANA-FREE SMOOTHIE

I've received a lot of requests for banana-free smoothies. It's a tall order within the context of a GP-friendly diet but it led me to this tasty concoction! It is fairly thick and filling, so you may need to add more water and/or turn it into two servings.

Ingredients

- 4 oz coconut milk
- 2-4 oz water
- 1/2 medium baked sweet potato, no peel
- 1 handful baby spinach
- 1 to 2 Tbsp pecan butter (or other nut/seed butter)
- 2 tsp maple syrup
- 1/2 to 1 tsp cinnamon

Directions

1. Put all ingredients in the blender, starting with milk.
2. Blend until creamy.
3. Enjoy!

SWEET-BANANA SMOOTHIE

This smoothie is a good reason to always have baked sweet potatoes in the fridge! You can eat this for breakfast with a scoop of nut butter for added fat and protein, or for dessert as a low-fat pumpkin "milkshake" without.

Ingredients

- 6 oz almond or coconut milk
- 1/2 banana, sliced and frozen
- 1/2 medium sweet potato, baked, and peeled
- 1/4 tsp vanilla extract
- 1/4 tsp cinnamon
- 1 Tbsp nut butter, optional

Directions

1. Add all ingredients to the blender, starting with liquid.
2. Blend until smooth, adding more liquid as necessary to reach desired consistency.

ALMOND JOY SMOOTHIE

"Sometimes you feel like a nut..." The chocolate flavor of this smoothie makes it seem like a dessert but add a scoop of protein powder and call it breakfast! **Not low-FOD-MAP due to cocoa powder.**

Ingredients

- 6 oz coconut milk, preferably homemade
- 1 Tbsp unsweetened cocoa powder
- 1 Tbsp almond butter
- 1 banana, frozen
- 2 tsp maple syrup (optional)
- 1 dash cinnamon

Directions

1. Add all ingredients to the blender, starting with liquid.
2. Blend until smooth, adding more liquid as necessary to reach desired consistency.

White Sweet Potato & Roasted Banana Puree

This tasty puree works for any meal of the day, even dessert! Orange sweet potatoes won't provide the same flavor, so be sure to use Jersey White. The nut butter is optional but recommended. Macadamias are rich in Omega 3s and may help reduce anxiety.

Ingredients

- 3 Jersey White sweet potatoes
- 2 bananas (peel on)
- 2 Tbsp macadamia nut butter, optional
- water, coconut milk, or almond milk

Directions

1. Preheat oven to 400°F.
2. Place whole sweet potatoes in a baking dish lined with parchment paper. Bake for 40 minutes.
3. Place bananas, peel on, into the dish and bake an additional 15 minutes.
4. Allow sweet potatoes and bananas to cool slightly.
5. Remove peels and skins.
6. Process in a food processor or blender, adding nut butter if desired and liquid as needed to achieve desired consistency.

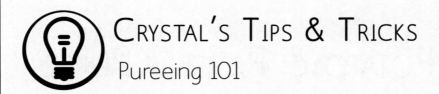

Crystal's Tips & Tricks
Pureeing 101

Tools

- ☐ collapsible mesh steamer and a medium sauce pot
- ☐ hand-turned food mill, food processor, blender, or Vitamix
- ☐ measuring cups
- ☐ freezer-safe Ziplock bags and/or freezer-safe storage containers

Steps

1. Prepare fruits and vegetables by washing, peeling, and chopping.

2. Cook fruits/vegetables, either by steaming, baking, or boiling until soft. If preparing a variety of purees, cook each separately.

3. Drain excess liquid then place cooked produce in food processor or blender and puree until smooth. You may need to add water or broth to achieve a smooth texture and/or a thinner consistency.

5. Cool purees. Measure into ½ cup portions and package in Ziplock bags or small food storage containers.

7. Store purees in the refrigerator if you'll be using them within 2-3 days, otherwise stick them in the freezer where they'll last for months.

Notes

- All frozen produce can be steamed frozen; no need to thaw.
- Sweet potatoes can be baked whole in the oven or a slow cooker until fork tender. Scoop out the flesh and puree.
- Leafy greens can be steamed or sautéed in a small amount of oil and then pureed. This will add a little healthy fat and improve the absorption of the fat soluble vitamins in your greens.

POTATO & PARSNIP PUREE

I first tried parsnips a few years ago and they have quickly become one of my favorite root vegetables. The flavor is similar to a carrot, though a bit more "woodsy." I think they pair really well with white potatoes, especially for purees.

Ingredients

- 1 lb parsnips
- 1-1/2 lbs white potatoes
- 1/2 to 1 cup chicken or vegetable broth
- sea salt, to taste

Directions

1. Peel and chop potatoes and parsnips.
2. Place in a saucepan. Cover with water and boil until soft, about 30 minutes.
3. Pass potatoes and parsnips through a potato ricer or food mill.
4. Stir in broth to achieve desired consistency.
5. Salt to taste.

Carrot &
Sweet Potato Puree

This naturally sweet puree offers a healthy dose of vitamins A and C. If you're not sensitive to FODMAPs, you can add applesauce instead of chicken broth to thin the mixture and add an extra hint of sweetness.

Ingredients

- 1-1/2 lbs carrots
- 1 lb sweet potatoes
- 1 cup chicken broth
- sea salt, to taste

Directions

1. Peel and chop carrots and sweet potatoes.
2. Place in a saucepan and cover with water.
3. Boil for 30 minutes or until soft.
4. Drain.
5. Pour veggies into a blender or food processor and puree, adding broth to thin to desired consistency.
6. Season to taste.

Gingered Squash Puree

*While butternut squash is fibrous, it's often well tolerated when pureed. This dish combines the nutritional benefits of squash with the anti-emetic properties of ginger. If you don't have fresh ginger, use ½-1 tsp of ground ginger. Portions larger than 1/4 cup are **not low-FODMAP.***

Ingredients

- 2 medium butternut squash
- 1 Tbsp butter or coconut oil
- 1 Tbsp maple syrup
- 1 to 2 Tbsp fresh ginger, finely grated (to taste)

- 3/4 tsp salt
- 1/8 tsp ground nutmeg

Directions

1. Preheat oven to 350°F.
2. Cut squash in half length-wise. Scoop out seeds.
3. Place halves cut-side down in a roasting pan. Add water to the pan to a depth of 1-inch.
4. Bake squash for 40-50 minutes, until easily pierced by a fork.
5. Cool squash. Scoop out the flesh and add to a food processor.
6. Add butter/oil and maple syrup. Process until smooth.
7. Add in ginger, salt, and nutmeg. Process until well blended, adding water if necessary to achieve desired consistency.
8. Serve immediately.

Maple Apple Pear Sauce

For a twist on regular applesauce, try this naturally sweetened fruit puree. It makes a tasty side dish, dessert, or snack. **Not low-FODMAP.**

Ingredients

- 4 medium apples, peeled and coarsely chopped
- 1 medium pear, peeled and coarsely chopped
- 3/4 cup water
- 1 Tbsp maple syrup, optional
- 1/2 tsp ground cinnamon
- 1/4 tsp ground nutmeg

Directions

1. Combine apples, pear, and water in a large saucepan over medium-high heat.
2. Bring to a boil. Reduce heat to a simmer.
3. Cover and cook 15-20 minutes or until very tender, stirring occasionally.
4. Add spices and maple syrup to taste. Mash with a potato masher or puree in food processor until desired consistency.
5. Serve warm or cold.

GREEN PEA PUREE

Mint pairs really well peas and can help to calm an upset stomach. If you don't toler-ate mint or you have been diagnosed with GERD, substitute parsley instead. **Peas are not low-FODMAP in servings greater than 1/4 cup.**

Ingredients

- 8 oz frozen peas
- 2 to 4 Tbsp chicken or vegetable broth
- 1 Tbsp chopped fresh mint or parsley
- sea salt, to taste

Directions

1. Steam peas until soft.
2. Add all ingredients to a blender and puree until smooth, adding more broth if necessary.

SOUPS

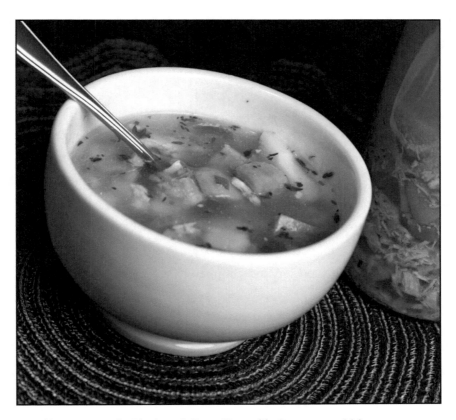

Totally Homemade Chicken & Root Vegetable Soup, page 116

WINTER VEGETABLE SOUP

This is one of the first recipes I created for myself when I started to understand that increasing nutrition was just as important as decreasing fat and fiber. It's still one of my favorites!

Ingredients

- 6 cups chicken or vegetable broth
- 1 tsp olive oil
- 1/4 cup green onions, chopped (green part only)
- 1/2 lb carrots, peeled and chopped
- 1 large parsnip, peeled and chopped
- 2 small turnips, peeled and chopped
- 3 medium potatoes, peeled and chopped
- 1/2-inch piece of fresh ginger, peeled
- 1 bay leaf
- 1 tsp sea salt

Directions

1. Heat olive oil in a large pot over medium-low heat. Add onions and cook two minutes.
2. Add all remaining ingredients.
3. Bring to a boil. Reduce heat and simmer at least 30 minutes, until veggies are very soft.
4. Fish out the bay leaf and ginger.
5. Puree the soup in a food processor or immersion blender until smooth. Add more broth, if necessary, to achieve desired consistency.

BEEF & VEGETABLE SOUP

Lean ground beef is a good source of iron and often well tolerated, however any ground meat or poultry can be used in this recipe. Bison or venison would be great! The buckwheat only adds about 1 gram of fiber per serving but it can easily be omitted.

Ingredients

- 2 tsp coconut oil
- 1 lb lean ground beef
- 6 cups vegetable stock
- 1 tsp sea salt
- 1 tsp dried parsley
- 1 tsp dried thyme
- 4 carrots, peeled and chopped
- 2 potatoes, peeled and chopped
- 1/3 cup soaked, uncooked buckwheat

Directions

1. Melt oil in a large pot over medium heat.
2. Add beef and cook until brown. Drain fat.
3. Add stock and spices. Bring to a boil then reduce to a simmer.
4. Add carrots, potatoes, and buckwheat and let simmer for about 30 minutes, until veggies are tender and buckwheat is cooked.

TOTALLY HOMEMADE CHICKEN & ROOT VEGETABLE SOUP

I've made this soup for many friends, from new moms to sick kids. Everyone loves it! The most time consuming part is making the broth but don't skip it! Homemade bone broth is what makes this soup so nourishing. If you already have 10-12 cups of home-made broth on hand, start with step 13 and add one pound cooked, chopped chicken breast along with the veggies and the spices

Ingredients

- 1 whole chicken, organic
- 14-16 cups of water
- 2 Tbsp apple cider vinegar
- 3 carrots
- 1 parsnip
- 1 medium sweet potato or 2 medium white potatoes
- 1/4 cup chopped green onions (green part only)
- 2-inch piece of ginger, peeled
- 1-2 tsp sea salt
- 1 tsp thyme
- 1/4 tsp basil
- 1/4 tsp oregano

Directions

1. Place chicken in a large stock pot and cover with water.
2. Slowly bring to a boil over medium heat. Skim off and discard the foam and fat that comes to the top.
3. Reduce heat and allow to gently boil for 1-1/2 to 2 hours, adding more liquid as necessary to keep the chicken covered.
4. Carefully remove the chicken and allow it to cool slightly. **Do not** discard the water.

Totally Homemade
Chicken & Root Vegetable Soup

Directions (continued)

5. Separate the meat from the bones. Discard skin. Reserve meat to be added back to the soup.

6. Put all of the bones back into stockpot. Add vinegar and allow to sit for 30 minutes before proceeding.

7. You can now transfer the broth to a preheated slow cooker or continue to boil on the stove.

8. Simmer either on the stove or in a slow cooker set on low for 6-20 more hours. (I usually do all of this in the evening and leave it to simmer in the slow cooker for 12 hours over night).

9. Allow broth to cool slightly. In the meantime, peel and chop your carrots, parsnips, sweet potato and/or white potato. Shred or chop the chicken meat you reserved.

10. Once broth has cooled down remove bones.

11. Strain broth through cheesecloth or a nut milk bag.

12. Skim off visible fat with a ladle or refrigerate the broth for 8 hours and skim all solidified fat off the top.

13. Add broth, chopped veggies, chicken meat, and spices to the pot. Bring to a gentle boil and cook until the veggies are soft, about 40 minutes.

14. Remove ginger. Let cool and transfer into jars. Store in the fridge for 4-5 days or freeze in individual portions.

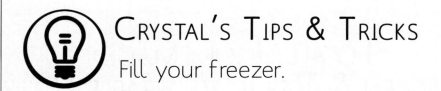

CRYSTAL'S TIPS & TRICKS
Fill your freezer.

When you're not feeling well, having a freezer stocked with home-made, nutrient-rich food for yourself and/or your family can be a saving grace. Stocking your freezer requires an initial time investment, but in the long run it will save you both time and energy. I recommend recruiting a friend or family member to help on prep day. You can also simply make double batches of foods that you cook often, such as grains, soups, and purees, sticking half in the freezer for another time.

Here are some of my favorite things to keep on hand in the freezer:

- cooked grains, including quinoa, buckwheat, and white rice
- cooked ground meats, including turkey, beef, and chicken
- individual portions of soups or stews
- smoothies
- fruit and vegetable juices (freeze in ice cube trays)
- fruit and vegetable purees (Infantino pouches freeze well)
- slow cooker meals (put uncooked meat, spices, chopped veg-gies, etc. in a freezer bag; when ready to cook just dump it in and set the slow cooker)

Be sure to cool food completely before freezing and store in freezer-safe containers. If you're freezing liquids, leave about an inch of space at the top of the container for expansion.

To reheat, thaw first in the refrigerator or pop right into the oven if you've stored the food in an oven-safe container.

CARROT & GINGER BISQUE

This is one of my favorite soups. Flavorful, satisfying, and nutrient-rich. A little bit of nutmeg goes a long way, so add just a bit at a time and taste test. This soup is relatively low in protein. Pair it with the Herbed Cod on page 133 for a tasty, balanced meal.

Ingredients

- 2 tsp red palm oil
- 1 shallot, chopped, optional
- 3 Tbsp finely chopped fresh ginger root
- 1 lb carrots, peeled and chopped
- 1 medium potato, peeled and chopped
- 6 cups chicken or vegetable stock
- 1 tsp sea salt
- dash nutmeg

Directions

1. Heat the oil in a large pot over medium heat.
2. Add the shallot and ginger. Sauté until shallot is translucent.
3. Add the carrots, potato and stock. Bring to a boil.
4. Cover, reduce heat and simmer until the vegetables are very tender, about 35-40 minutes.
5. Purée in a food processor or with an immersion blender.
6. Add salt and nutmeg.

TURKEY SOUP

This is a great use of leftover Slow Cooker Turkey Breast (page 128). It's also great for holidays, especially if you're not able to tolerate a traditional turkey dinner. If you don't have turkey broth, use chicken or vegetable broth instead.

Ingredients

- 6 cups turkey broth
- 2 cups chopped cooked skinless turkey breast
- 1 large celery rib, cut in half
- 1/4 cup green onions, finely chopped (green parts only)
- 1-1/2 tsp sea salt
- 1/2 tsp dried marjoram
- 2 bay leaves
- 3 medium potatoes, peeled and chopped
- 6 large carrots, peeled and sliced

Directions

1. Combine all ingredients in a large pot.
2. Bring to a boil. Reduce heat to a simmer.
3. Simmer for 40 minutes or until veggies are tender.
4. Remove from heat. Carefully remove bay leaf and celery stalks before serving.

Chicken Noodle Soup

This is my gluten-free, FODMAP-friendly twist on the classic "feel good" soup. The egg noodles can be replaced with any brown rice or quinoa pasta.

Ingredients

- 2 tsp butter or olive oil
- 4 carrots, peeled and chopped
- 1/2 cup green onions, chopped (green part only)
- 2 potatoes, peeled and diced
- 1 tsp thyme
- 1 bay leaf
- 8 cups chicken broth
- 6 oz gluten-free egg noodles
- 2 cups cooked chicken breast, chopped
- 1/2 to 1 tsp sea salt, to taste

Directions

1. Melt butter or heat oil in large pot.
2. Sauté the carrots and onions for 2-3 minutes.
3. Add potatoes, thyme, bay leaf, and chicken broth.
4. Bring to a boil.
5. Add noodles and chicken.
6. Reduce heat and simmer for 20 minutes, until noodles are cooked and veggies are tender.
7. Salt to taste.

VEGETABLE SOUP

Though this soup calls for some higher-fiber (and less common) root veggies, the finished product is still GP-friendly with one cup containing about three grams of fiber. If you're following a soft food diet, this soup also tastes delicious pureed.

Ingredients

- 2 tsp olive oil
- 1/2 cup green onions, chopped (green part only)
- 2 carrots, peeled and chopped
- 1 parsnip, peeled and chopped
- 1 rutabaga, peeled and chopped
- 1 turnip, peeled and chopped
- 2 bay leaves
- 2 Tbsp fresh parsley, chopped
- 6 cups vegetable broth
- sea salt, to taste

Directions

1. Heat oil over medium-low in a large stock pot. Add green onions and cook two minutes.
2. Add all other ingredients. Bring to a boil.
3. Reduce heat to a simmer. Cook 20-30 minutes, until the veggies are soft.
4. Season to taste.

MAIN DISHES

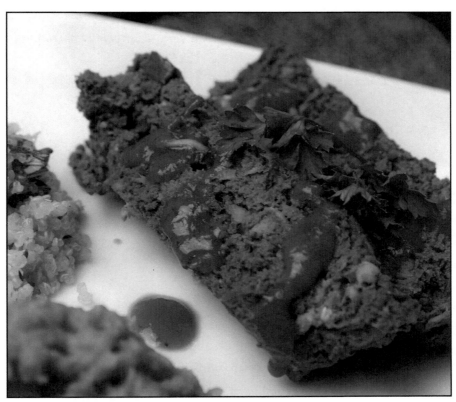

Tomato-Less Meatloaf, page 131

ROASTED CHICKEN & ROOT VEGETABLES

This is my most requested recipe. It's absolutely delicious and really simple. I use skin-on bone-in chicken breasts for two reasons: the skin keeps the meat moist and I save the bones to make chicken stock. GPers should remove the chicken skin before eating.

Ingredients

- 6 carrots, peeled and chopped
- 3 white potatoes, peeled and chopped
- 2 medium sweet potatoes, peeled and chopped
- 2 Tbsp coconut oil or red palm oil
- 1 tsp sea salt
- 1 tsp dried thyme
- 3 lb bone-in chicken breasts

Directions

1. Preheat oven to 375°F. If oil is solid, place it into a large baking dish and put it in the oven while it preheats.
2. Peel and chop all vegetables.
3. Add vegetables to the baking dish, stirring to coat in oil.
4. Place chicken breasts in the center of the baking dish.
5. Sprinkle chicken and vegetables with sea salt and thyme.
6. Roast for 50-60 minutes, until chicken has reached an internal temperature of 160 degrees and vegetables are fork tender and slightly browned.

OVEN "FRIED" CHICKEN

While you could use a gluten-free biscuit mix or all-purpose flour for this recipe, I don't see the need for the "gums" and leaveners that are typically added to those mixes. A simple one-ingredient rice flour works!

Ingredients

- 2 lbs skinless chicken breast
- 2/3 cup brown rice flour
- 1/2 tsp paprika
- 1 tsp sea salt
- 1 Tbsp butter or red palm oil

Directions

1. Preheat oven to 425°F.
2. Spoon butter or oil into a 13 x 9- inch baking dish and put it in the oven while it's preheating.
3. Combine flour, paprika, and salt in a gallon size Ziplock bag.
4. Add 1 piece of chicken at a time to the Ziplock bag and shake well to coat.
5. Put the coated chicken into the buttered/oiled baking dish.
6. Bake for 20 minutes; turn pieces over and bake an additional 20 minutes or until internal temperature reaches 160°F.

THYME & LEMON CHICKEN WITH POTATOES

Green beans are not GP-friendly, so if you're making this just for you, leave them out and use 2 pounds of potatoes. I usually make it with the green beans so that I don't have to prepare an additional side for my family. This dish is great for company!

Ingredients

- 2 Tbsp coconut oil, melted
- juice of 1 lemon, about 1/4 cup
- 1 tsp sea salt
- 1 tsp dried thyme
- 1 lb green beans
- 1-1/2 lb potatoes, about 4 medium-sized
- 4 boneless, skinless chicken breasts (about 1-1/2 to 2 lbs)

Directions

1. Preheat oven to 425°F.
2. Wash and trim green beans. Peel and cube potatoes.
3. Combine oil, lemon juice, salt, and thyme in a large bowl.
4. Dredge green beans and potatoes through the oil mixture. Arrange along the outside of a large baking dish.
5. Dredge chicken through remaining oil mixture and place in the middle of the baking dish.
6. Roast for 40 minutes, stirring vegetables occasionally, until the internal temperature of the chicken reaches 165°F and the potatoes and green beans are soft and slightly browned.

QUICK TURKEY FRIED RICE

This is an easy throw-together lunch. You can even cook the meat in advance. The tumeric adds a nice flavor and is anti-inflammatory. Experiment with the veggies to find what you like and tolerate best. Peas are my current favorite!

Ingredients

- 2 tsp coconut oil
- 1 lb ground turkey breast
- 2 cups cooked rice
- 1 cup cooked diced vegetables
- 1 tsp sea salt
- 1 tsp tumeric

Directions

1. Melt coconut oil in a skillet over medium heat.
2. Add turkey and cook until no longer pink.
3. Add rice, vegetables, and spices.
4. Stir to combine and continue cooking until heated through, about three minutes.

SLOW COOKER TURKEY BREAST

Cooking this flavorful turkey breast is so much easier than preparing a whole turkey and because it's skinless and all white meat, it's all GP-friendly!

Ingredients

- 1 bone-in turkey breast (6 to 7 lbs), skin removed
- 1 Tbsp olive oil
- 1 tsp salt
- 1/2 tsp paprika
- 1/2 tsp thyme
- 1/2 tsp oregano

Directions

1. Brush turkey with oil.
2. Combine the remaining ingredients in a small bowl. Rub over turkey.
3. Transfer turkey to a 6-quart slow cooker.
4. Cover and cook on low for 6 hours or until internal temperature reaches 165°F.

SLOW COOKER BISON STEW

I've used both beef and bison in this recipe. I prefer bison as it's naturally lean and still quite flavorful. I tolerate peas so I include them. If you do not, add two more carrots instead. I usually serve this to others alongside a simple side salad.

Ingredients

- 1 lb bison (or beef) stew meat
- 4 carrots
- 2 medium white or sweet potatoes
- 1 cup frozen peas, optional
- 2 cups water
- 1 Tbsp tapioca starch
- 1-1/2 tsp thyme
- 1-1/2 tsp sea salt
- 1-1/2 tsp basil
- 1-1/2 tsp oregano

Directions

1. Peel and chop potatoes and carrots.
2. Add all ingredients to your slow cooker. Stir to combine.
3. Cook for 6-8 hours on Low.

Shepard's Pie

I've been making Shepard's Pie for my husband for years but never thought to create a GP-friendly version until recently. It's a simple, comforting one-dish meal. Add any additional vegetables that you tolerate, such as shredded zucchini or baby peas. If you tolerate dairy, add a sprinkle on top before baking to make it extra tasty!

Ingredients

- 1 tsp coconut oil
- 1 lb lean ground beef, ground bison, or ground venison
- 4 carrots, peeled and shredded
- 1-1/2 pounds white or sweet potatoes

- 1-1/2 cup beef stock, divided
- 1 Tbsp tapioca starch
- 1-1/2 tsp sea salt, divided
- 1/2 tsp thyme
- 1/4 tsp rosemary
- 1/4 tsp basil

Directions

1. Preheat oven to 350°F.
2. Melt oil in a skillet over medium heat. Cook meat. Drain fat.
3. Add 3/4 cup beef stock, 1/2 tsp salt, spices, and tapioca starch. Cook until thickened then remove from heat.
4. Peel and dice potatoes. Boil until soft. Drain.
5. Mash potatoes, adding remaining beef stock and 1 tsp salt.
6. In a 9-inch pie plate, layer beef mixture, shredded carrots, and mashed potatoes.
7. Bake for 30 minutes, until carrots are softened and the top is slightly browned.

TOMATO-LESS MEATLOAF

It's not easy to find a meatloaf recipe that's not laden with fat, FODMAPs, and to-matoes! It took some tinkering but this one is a winner. You can substitute any ground meat or poultry for the beef.

Ingredients

- 1 cup gluten-free rolled oats
- 7 oz roasted red peppers
- 1 lb lean ground beef
- 1/4 cup green onions, chopped very fine (green part only)
- 1 tsp basil
- 1 tsp oregano
- 1 tsp thyme
- 1 tsp sea salt

Directions

1. Preheat oven to 375°F. Line a rimmed baking sheet with foil.
2. Pulverize oats in a food processor until they are a coarse flour.
3. Puree roasted red peppers in a food processor or blender.
4. Combine all ingredients in a bowl.
5. Form mixture into a loaf shape and place it on baking sheet.
6. Bake for 50 minutes.
7. Let cool 5-10 minutes before slicing.

10-MINUTE SALMON

Salmon is a fantastic source of Omega-3 fatty acids, a common deficiency among GPers. My favorite is wild-caught silver salmon, which we purchase from www.VitalChoice.com. It is lower in fat and has a milder flavor than other varieties.

Ingredients

- 2 tsp coconut oil
- 4 pieces of salmon, about 5 oz each
- 1 tsp lemon zest
- 1 tsp thyme
- 1/2 tsp sea salt

Directions

1. Preheat oven to 500°F.
2. Rub coconut oil onto bottom of baking dish.
3. Place salmon skin side down in baking dish.
4. Combine lemon zest, thyme, and sea salt in small bowl.
5. Sprinkle evenly over salmon pieces.
6. Bake for 10 minutes or until internal temperature reaches 140-145°F. Do not overcook.

HERB-BAKED COD

Cod is a very low fat, mild tasting fish. It's a great source of protein and is typically well-tolerated by those with gastroparesis. Pair this with Confetti Millet (page 147) for an easy-to-prepare dinner that's fancy enough for company.

Ingredients

- 4- 5 oz pieces of cod
- 1 Tbsp olive oil
- 1 tsp sea salt
- 1/2 tsp rosemary
- 1/2 tsp thyme
- 1/2 tsp basil

Directions

1. Preheat oven to 350°F.
2. Place cod on a parchment-lined baking sheet.
3. Combine oil and herbs in a small bowl.
4. Spread oil/herb mixture over fish.
5. Bake for about 15 minutes, or until it flakes easily with a fork and reaches an internal temperature of 145°F.

TILAPIA FLORENTINE

While citrus may trigger reflux, the amount of lemon juice per serving is quite small in this recipe and likely to be well-tolerated. If you'd rather omit the lemon juice, the recipe will still work.

Ingredients

- 4 tilapia filets (4 oz each)
- 1 (12 oz) bag cut leaf spinach
- 1 Tbsp coconut oil
- 1/2 lemon, juiced
- 1 teaspoon sea salt
- 1/2 tsp dried parsley
- Parmesan cheese, optional

Directions

1. Preheat oven to 375°F.
2. Spread frozen spinach on the bottom of a large baking dish.
3. Arrange fish fillets over top of the spinach.
4. In a small bowl, combine coconut oil, lemon juice, and spices.
5. Drizzle oil mixture over fish and spinach.
6. Cover and bake for 15 minutes.
7. Uncover and bake for an additional 15 minutes or until the internal temperature of the fish reaches 145°F.
8. Serve with a sprinkle of Parmesan cheese, if desired.

VEGGIES & SIDES

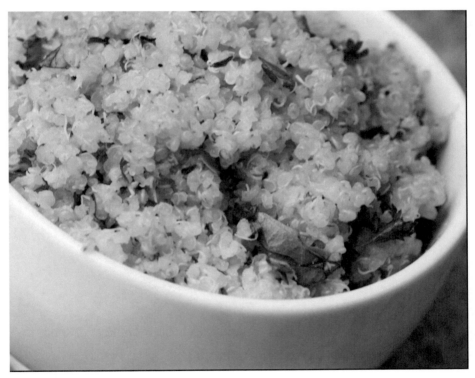

Basic Quinoa, page 147

LAZY BAKED SWEET POTATOES

This is more of a method than a recipe but every time I mention it on Facebook, there are many follow-up questions. This is how I cook sweet potatoes for mashing, pureeing, and making hash. It's easier than peeling/boiling and retains more nutrients, too.

Ingredients

- 3 lbs sweet potatoes

Directions

1. Place whole, unpeeled sweet potatoes in slow cooker. (No need for liquid or any other preparations.)
2. Cook on high for 3-1/2 hours, depending on your slow cooker, until easily pierced with a fork.

BALSAMIC ROASTED VEGGIES

Balsamic vinegar and walnut oil take simple roasted vegetables to the next level. Omit mushrooms for a low-FODMAP version. If you don't tolerate balsamic vinegar, simply roast the vegetables in oil.

Ingredients

- 1 large sweet potato, peeled and cubed
- 1/2 lb baking potatoes, peeled and cubed
- 1/2 lb carrots, peeled and thickly sliced
- 1/2 lb turnips, peeled and cubed
- 6 oz mushrooms, halved
- 1 Tbsp walnut oil
- 1/2 Tbsp balsamic vinegar
- 1 tsp sea salt

Directions

1. Preheat oven to 425°F.
2. In a large roasting pan, combine vegetables, oil, vinegar, and salt.
3. Roast for 35-40 minutes, or until vegetables are tender and lightly browned.
4. Serve warm or at room temperature.

CARROT CHIPS

These baked chips are surprisingly crispy and so much healthier than store bought veggie chips fried in low-quality oils. Perfect for a quick snack or a lunchtime side. (Don't under cook them or they'll be chewy.)

Ingredients

- 4 carrots
- 2 tsp coconut oil, melted
- sea salt, to taste

Directions

1. Preheat oven to 350°F.
2. Peel carrots.
3. Pressing hard with a vegetable peeler, peel long slices off of the carrots.
4. Toss with oil.
5. Arrange on a parchment lined baking sheet.
6. Sprinkle with salt.
7. Bake 15-20 minutes, turning once, until crispy.
8. Allow to cool before eating.

MASHED CAULIFLOWER

*Need a break from potatoes? Cauliflower makes excellent "faux" mashed potatoes. While cauliflower isn't GP-friendly whole or raw, it's often well tolerated when pureed. **Not low-FODMAP.***

Ingredients

- 1 head of cauliflower, florets only
- 1/2 cup chicken broth
- 1/4 cup grated Parmesan cheese, optional
- sea salt, to taste

Directions

1. Fill a medium pot with water and bring to a boil over high heat.
2. Add cauliflower florets and cook for 8–10 minutes or until soft.
3. Drain.
4. In a food processor, combine the cauliflower, 1/4 cup broth, and Parmesan cheese, if desired. Puree until creamy.
5. Add remaining chicken broth, a tablespoon at a time, until the desired consistency is reached.
6. Add salt to taste.

Parmesan Potato Fries

If you are not sensitivity to dairy, Parmesan cheese is a low-fat, low-lactose, low-FODMAP option. Use real Parmesan cheese with no fillers or additional ingredients for these tasty fries.

Ingredients

- 4 large baking potatoes, peeled
- 1 Tbsp olive oil
- 1/4 cup grated Parmesan cheese
- 1 tsp sea salt

Directions

1. Preheat oven to 425°F. Line a baking sheet with heavy-duty foil.
2. Cut each potato into thin french-fry shaped pieces.
3. Put potatoes, olive oil, Parmesan cheese and salt into a bowl and toss to coat.
4. Arrange in a single layer on baking sheet.
5. Bake for 30–40 minutes, flipping once, until tender inside and crispy outside.

ROSEMARY ROASTED CARROTS

This is a fancy-seeming but utterly simple side. Roasting carrots at a high temperature intensifies the natural sweetness, which pairs well with the savory rosemary. All or some of the roasted carrots can be pureed in a food processor, if a soft dish is desired.

Ingredients

- 1 lb carrots, peeled
- 2 tsp red palm or coconut oil
- 1 tsp dried rosemary
- 1/2 tsp sea salt

Directions

1. Preheat oven to 450°F.
2. Cut carrots into 1-inch pieces.
3. Toss carrots with oil, rosemary, and salt until well coated.
4. Place in a roasting pan.
5. Roast 30-35 minutes, until very soft and beginning to brown.

ROASTED RED PEPPER MASHED POTATOES

Eating food in a rainbow of colors each day is a simple way to enhance variety and overall nutrition in a GP-friendly diet. This family-friendly recipe adds some "red" to a GP-friendly staple, mashed potatoes. Boil the potatoes on the stove if you prefer.

Ingredients

- 3 lbs organic white potatoes
- 1-1/2 to 2 cups chicken broth, divided
- 2 large roasted red peppers
- 1 tsp sea salt
- 1 Tbsp butter or red palm oil, optional

Directions

1. Peel and chop potatoes into small chunks.
2. Place potatoes and 1 cup of chicken broth into slow cooker.
3. Cover and cook on high for 4 hours or until potatoes are tender.
4. Heat remaining chicken broth. Add 1/2 cup to cooked potatoes and mash to desired consistency, adding additional broth as necessary. Stir in butter, if desired.
5. Rinse and remove seeds from roasted red peppers.
6. Puree peppers in a food processor or blender until smooth.
7. Stir red pepper puree and salt into mashed potatoes until combined.

ROASTED ACORN SQUASH

This side dish quickly becomes an all-in-one meal if you fill the cavity with cooked and seasoned ground meat after baking. Ground pork with sage and another drizzle of maple syrup is one of my faves!

Ingredients

- 2 acorn squash
- 4 tsp coconut oil
- 4 tsp maple syrup
- 1/2 tsp cinnamon
- 1/4 tsp sea salt

Directions

1. Preheat oven to 400°F
2. Wash squash and cut each in half lengthwise. Scoop out seeds.
3. Place skin side down in a baking dish.
4. Rub cut side of each half with 1 teaspoon coconut oil.
5. Drizzle each half with 1 teaspoon maple syrup.
6. Sprinkle each half with cinnamon and salt.
7. Roast in the oven for 45 to 60 minutes, until fork tender.
8. Eat as is, avoiding the skin, or scoop flesh into a blender and puree.

CREAMY MASHED POTATOES

Chicken stock takes the place of cream and butter in this simple yet satisfying mashed potato recipe. For the yummiest, most nourishing potatoes, use homemade stock!

Ingredients

- 4 large white potatoes (about 1-1/2 lbs)
- 8 oz chicken broth, warmed
- sea salt, to taste

Directions

1. Peel and dice potatoes.
2. Boil potatoes until tender. Drain well.
3. Mash or put through a potato ricer, adding broth until desired consistency is reached.
4. Season to taste.

WHIPPED SWEET POTATOES

I like the added flavor and hint of sweetness from the orange juice and don't find that irritates my stomach but you can substitute 1/2 cup of any liquid if you do not tolerate citrus.

Ingredients

- 3 lbs organic sweet potatoes
- 1/4 cup fresh squeezed orange juice
- 1/4 cup water
- 1-1/2 Tbsp coconut oil
- 1-1/2 tsp cinnamon
- 1 tsp sea salt

Directions

1. Preheat oven to 375°F.
2. Place whole, unpeeled sweet potatoes in a parchment-lined baking dish (for easier clean-up!).
3. Bake for 45-60 minutes, until a fork easily pierces them.
4. Allow to sit until cool enough to handle. Slice each in half and scoop out the inside with a spoon. Discard peels.
5. Add the sweet potato flesh and all ingredients to a blender or food processor and whip until smooth.

TUMERIC RICE

Turmeric is a brightly-colored spice with powerful anti-inflammatory properties. Omit the mushrooms if you're following a low-FODMAP diet.

Ingredients

- 2 tsp olive oil
- 2 cups chicken broth
- 1 cup basmati or jasmine rice
- 1/2 cup thinly sliced mushrooms
- 1/2 tsp turmeric
- sea salt, to taste

Directions

1. Rinse the rice in a fine mesh strainer under cold water until water runs clear. Place rice in a large bowl, cover with water and let sit for 30 minutes before proceeding with the recipe.
2. Heat oil in a medium saucepan over medium heat. Add rice and sauté for 2 minutes, stirring frequently.
3. Add broth, mushrooms, and turmeric. Increase heat and bring to a boil.
4. Reduce heat to low. Cover and simmer for 18–20 minutes, until broth is absorbed and rice is tender.
5. Fluff with a fork before serving. Add salt to taste.

BASIC QUINOA

Quinoa is an ancient grain-like seed that is relatively high in protein and often-well tolerated by those with gastroparesis. Cooking the quinoa in homemade broth increases both the flavor and nutrition. To make this recipe vegan, simply substitute vegetable broth. There are 4 grams of fiber per 1/2 cup of cooked quinoa, so stick to one serving.

Ingredients

- 1 cup uncooked quinoa, soaked or sprouted
- 2 cups chicken broth
- 1/2 tsp sea salt
- 1 Tbsp olive oil, optional
- 2-3 Tbsp finely chopped fresh thyme and/or parsley, optional

Directions

1. Bring quinoa, broth, and salt to a boil over high heat.
2. Reduce heat, cover, and simmer for 15 minutes.
3. Remove from heat and allow to rest, covered, for 5 minutes.
4. Fluff with a fork. Add optional ingredients, if desired.

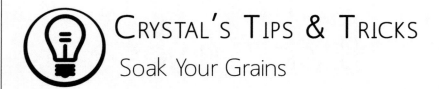

CRYSTAL'S TIPS & TRICKS
Soak Your Grains

Why soak grains?

All grains contain an anti-nutrient called phytic acid, which prevents the body from absorbing important minerals such as calcium, zinc, iron, phosphorous, and magnesium. Phytic acid not only impairs nutrient absorption, it also inhibits digestive enzymes that we need to break down our food, including pepsin, amylase, and trypsin. Together, this may contribute to digestive symptoms, as well as further nutrient deficiencies.

In traditional cultures, grains were soaked, soured, or sprouted prior to cooking. A combination of soaking grains in an acidic solution and then cooking them is the best way to break down phytic acid and make grains easier to digest. Small amounts of soaked and cooked grains, including buckwheat, millet, and quinoa, may be well-tolerated as part of a gastroparesis-friendly diet.

Directions

1. Place uncooked whole grains into a bowl. Cover with warm water.
2. Add 1 Tbsp apple cider vinegar or lemon juice per cup of grains.
3. Place the bowl in a warm location (an unheated oven with the light on will work) and soak for 8-24 hours. (Soak buckwheat just 7 hours to avoid a mushy consistency.)
4. Drain water and rinse very well.
5. Cook as directed, decreasing cooking time slightly to account for soaking.

CONFETTI MILLET

Millet can be rather bland on it's own but this recipe really jazzes it up with root veggies and chives. If you're not a fan of chives, you can substitute green onions (or shallot if you're not on a low-FODMAP diet).

Ingredients

- 1 tsp coconut oil
- 1 cup uncooked millet, soaked
- 3 cups chicken
- 3 carrots
- 2 parsnips
- 2 Tbsp finely chopped chives
- 1/2 tsp sea salt

Directions

1. Peel carrots and parsnips. Chop very fine or pulse in a food processor until finely chopped.
2. Melt oil in a medium pot over low heat. Add millet and toast 2 minutes, stirring often.
3. Add all other ingredients to the pot.
4. Bring to a boil. Reduce heat to a simmer.
5. Cover and simmer for 25-30 minutes, until broth is absorbed.
6. Let stand 5 minutes. Fluff with a fork before serving.

CHEATER RISOTTO

Making traditional risotto requires a lot of time and stirring. This GP-friendly version is much easier. Parmesan is a low-fat, low-lactose cheese that is often well-tolerated by those who are not sensitive to dairy. Be sure to use the real thing!

Ingredients

- 2 tsp butter or olive oil
- 2/3 cup uncooked Arborio rice
- 2 cups chicken broth, divided
- 1/4 cup grated Parmesan cheese (not "shake cheese")
- 1/2 tsp sea salt

Directions

1. Melt butter or heat oil in a medium saucepan over medium heat. Add rice and cook for 2 minutes, stirring frequently.
2. Add 1-3/4 cups of the broth. Bring to a boil.
3. Reduce heat and simmer, covered, for 20 minutes.
4. Remove saucepan from heat and let stand, covered, for 5 minutes.
5. Add remaining broth, Parmesan cheese, and salt. Stir very well.

TREATS

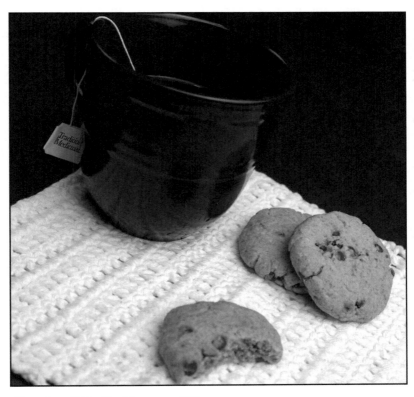

Chocolate Chip Cookies, page 153

OATMEAL CHOCOLATE CHUNK COOKIES

Between my toddler's dairy, egg, and nut allergies and my gluten intolerance it took me a while to come up with a cookie recipe that didn't require multiple flours and starches. It was worth the trial-and-error! These are delicious and so easy to make.

Ingredients

- 3 cups gluten-free oats
- 1/2 cup palm oil
- 1/4 cup unrefined coconut oil
- 1/3 cup maple syrup
- 1/3 cup sucanat or brown sugar
- 2 tsp vanilla extract
- 1 tsp baking powder
- 1/3 cup chocolate chips

Directions

1. Preheat oven to 375°F. Line a baking sheet with parchment paper.
2. Process oats in a food processor or high-speed blender until it becomes flour.
3. In a mixing bowl, cream oils, sucanat, maple syrup, and vanilla until fluffy, about 1 minute.
4. Add oat flour and baking powder. Mix until combined.
5. Fold in chocolate chips.
6. Scoop by the tablespoon onto the baking sheet.
7. Bake for 10 minutes. Cool completely before removing from the cookie sheet to avoid crumbling.

CHOCOLATE CHIP COOKIES

Don't be put off by the long ingredient list. It's worth it! These cookies taste just like the "real thing" even though they're vegan and gluten-free.. Each cookie has about 5 grams of fat so limit yourself to one per sitting.

Ingredients

- 1-1/4 cup sorghum flour
- 1/2 cup brown rice flour
- 1/4 cup millet flour
- 3/4 cup potato starch
- 3/4 cup tapioca flour
- 1-1/2 tsp xanthan gum
- 1-1/2 tsp baking soda
- 1 tsp baking powder
- 1 tsp sea salt
- 1 cup palm shortening
- 3 Tbsp coconut oil
- 1/2 cup maple syrup
- 1/2 cup brown sugar
- 1/2 cup sugar
- 1 Tbsp vanilla extract
- 1 cup Enjoy Life mini-chocolate chips

Directions

1. Preheat oven to 350°F.
2. Combine dry ingredients in a medium bowl.
3. In a large mixing bowl, beat shortening and oil until combined.
4. Add maple syrup, sugars, and vanilla. Beat 2 minutes.
5. Gradually add dry ingredients to wet ingredients. Mix until combined. Stir in chocolate chips.
6. Scoop by the tablespoon onto parchment lined baking sheets. Flatten tops with a spoon (they will not spread during baking).
7. Bake for 11-12 minutes. Transfer to wire rack to cool.

BIRTHDAY CUPCAKES

For many years after my GP diagnosis, I didn't have a birthday cake. These days, we make these GP-friendly (gluten-free, vegan) cupcakes for my birthday and everyone else's! Each cupcake has about 2.5 grams of fat each.

Ingredients

- 1 cup sorghum flour
- 1 cup tapioca starch
- 1 tsp baking powder
- 1 tsp baking soda
- 1 tsp xanthan gum
- 1/2 tsp sea salt

- 3 Tbsp coconut oil, softened
- 1 cup raw cane sugar
- 1 cup light coconut milk
- 1/4 cup applesauce
- 1 Tbsp vanilla extract
- Light Chocolate Frosting, page 155

Directions

1. Preheat oven to 350°F. Line a muffin tin with cupcake liners.
2. Mix all dry ingredients (except sugar) in a medium bowl.
3. Beat coconut oil and sugar in a mixing bowl. Slowly beat in milk. Add applesauce and vanilla. Mix to combine.
4. Add dry ingredients to wet ingredients and beat for 1-2 minutes, until fluffy.
5. Scoop by the 1/4 cup into muffin liners.
6. Bake for 20 minutes. Cool completely before frosting.

LIGHT CHOCOLATE FROSTING

This isn't bakery-style fluffy, sugary frosting... but it's low-fat, chocolatey, and tastes pretty darn good on my Birthday Cupcakes. The frosting, divided evenly between 12 cupcakes, will add about 2.5 grams of fat per cupcake (a total of 5 grams each).

Ingredients

- 1 banana
- 2 Tbsp cocoa powder
- 2 Tbsp palm oil shortening
- 1 cup powdered sugar
- 1 tsp vanilla extract

Directions

1. Puree banana.
2. Whip banana and palm oil shortening with an electric mixer.
3. Add in cocoa powder, powdered sugar, and vanilla.
4. Beat until fluffy, adding nondairy milk to thin to desired consistency.

Notes

This recipe is **not low-FODMAP** due to the cocoa powder. As an alternative, replace the palm oil shortening with peanut butter and omit the cocoa powder. This version is also lower in fat, about 1.3 grams per serving.

IN-A-PINCH BROWNIES

I don't advocate including many boxed foods in your diet, especially treats. But once in a while you need brownies in a hurry, whether for unexpected guests or a last minute potluck. No one will know these are GP-friendly, dairy-free, and gluten-free. Promise!

Ingredients

- 1 (16 oz) box Betty Crocker Gluten Free Brownie Mix
- 1/2 cup unsweetened applesauce
- 1 egg
- 1/4 cup water

Directions

1. Preheat oven to 350°F. Line the bottom of a 9 x 9-inch pan with parchment paper.
2. Combine all ingredients in a bowl and stir until just combined. Don't over mix.
3. Pour into prepared pan and bake for 30–32 minutes, until a toothpick inserted 2 inches from the edge comes out clean. Do not over bake.
4. Cool before cutting.

BETTER RICE CRISPY BARS

Rice Krispie Treats tend to be well-tolerated but the traditional recipe is loaded with processed ingredients. This makeover is a bit higher in fat -- watch your portions! -- but better nutritionally. Brown rice syrup can be found online and in many supermarkets.

Ingredients

- 1/2 cup creamy nut or seed butter (sunflower, peanut, almond)
- 1/2 cup brown rice syrup
- 1 tsp vanilla extract
- 4 cups puffed rice cereal (e.g. Erewhon's)

Directions

1. Line a 9 x 9-inch baking dish with parchment paper.
2. Measure cereal into a large bowl.
3. In a medium saucepan, combine nut butter, brown rice syrup, and vanilla extract. Stir over low heat until well combined.
4. Pour mixture over cereal and stir well to coat.
5. Spread mixture into prepared dish.
6. Refrigerate for one hour before cutting.

BANANA ICE CREAM

This is barely a recipe... there's only one required ingredient! But the idea is genius and so perfect for those on a whole-food, GP-friendly diet. Start with the basic version and then get creative with add-ins to find your favorite flavor.

Ingredients

- 2 bananas, chunked and frozen

Optional Add-Ins

- 1 Tbsp unsweetened cocoa powder (not low-FODMAP)
- 2 Tbsp peanut, almond, or sunflower seed butter

Directions

1. Place frozen banana chunks in a food processor.
2. Process until small pebbles form.
3. Wipe down the bowl and continue to process until mixture becomes light and fluffy, similar to the consistency of soft serve, ice cream.
4. Add optional ingredients and pulse to combine.
5. Enjoy immediately.

BANANA MUFFINS

These are gluten-free, vegan, and nut-free. Though they're low-fat as far as muffins go, each one still has about five grams of fat so stick to one serving! If you tolerate chocolate and a little extra fat, a 1/4 cup chocolate chips makes a nice addition.

Ingredients

- 1 cup sorghum flour
- 1/4 cup tapioca starch
- 1/4 cup potato starch
- 1/2 tsp xanthan gum
- 1 tsp baking powder
- ½ tsp baking soda
- ½ tsp sea salt

- 2 large ripe bananas, mashed
- 1/4 cup coconut oil, melted
- 1/2 cup pure maple syrup
- 1 tsp vanilla
- 1/4 cup Enjoy Life mini chocolate chips, optional

Directions

1. Preheat oven to 350°F.
2. Combine dry ingredients in a medium bowl.
3. In a blender combine bananas, oil, maple syrup and bananas.
4. Stir wet ingredients into dry ingredients until combined.
5. Add chocolate chips if desired.
6. Bake for 18-20 minutes or until the center of the muffins read 190°F on a digital thermometer.

SLOW COOKER RICE PUDDING

Put this in the slow cooker before dinner and in a couple of hours you'll have a warm, comforting dessert. Use any kind of nondairy milk that you tolerate.

Ingredients

- 3/4 cup short-grain rice
- 1-1/2 cups almond milk
- 2 cups water
- 3/4 cup maple syrup
- 1-1/2 tsp vanilla
- 1 tsp ground cinnamon

Directions

1. Combine all ingredients in slow cooker; stir well.
2. Cover and cook on "Low" for 4 to 5 hours or on "High" for 2 to 2-1/2 hours.
3. Stir twice during cooking process.
4. Serve warm.

Mexican Hot Cocoa

*Sadly cocoa powder is **not low FODMAP,** but if you can tolerate it this is a wonderful treat on a cold night. Or any night... I drank it all through my summer pregnancy!*

Ingredients

- 1 1/2 cups of unsweetened almond milk
- 2 Tbsp cocoa powder
- 2-1/2 Tbsp sugar
- 1/4 tsp ground cinnamon
- 1/2 tsp vanilla extract

Directions

1. In a small saucepan, combine cocoa powder, sugar, and cinnamon.
2. Stirring constantly, add milk and heat over medium heat until hot — but do not boil.
3. Remove from heat. Stir in 1/2 tsp vanilla extract.
4. Serve immediately.

PART FOUR:
DAY-TO-DAY CONCERNS

Hopefully this book has alleviated your confusion and frustration about what and how to eat after a gastroparesis diagnosis. By adhering to the guidelines set forth in Part One, the food list provided in Part Two, and the recipes offered in Part Three, you'll be well on your way to implementing your own version of the GP-friendly diet.

As we wrap up, I'd like to address some additional challenges that are related to following a gastroparesis-friendly diet beyond the basics of choosing and cooking your own food at home. You can find much more about each of these topics at www.LivingWithGastroparesis.com.

A printable version of the sample meal plan that follows can be found on the Book Resources page at www.EatingForGastroparesis.com. There you'll also find direct links to my favorite kitchen tools and products, my Amazon Subscribe & Save list, and my pantry staples as outlined in Parts Two and Three.

Sample 4-Day Meal Plan

Even with a firm grasp on the guidelines of a GP-friendly diet, it can be difficult to picture exactly what a day's worth of nutrient-rich meals looks like. Here I've created a sample 4-day meal plan using the recipes in Part Three.

Unless otherwise indicated, the meal plan is based on one serving of each recipe (page number in parentheses). Each day's menu contains *approximately* 12 to 15 grams of fiber and 30 to 40 grams of fat. To determine the exact nutritional information based on the ingredients you use and the quantity you eat, I recommend using www.MyFitnessPal.com. Please keep in mind that this is just an example of what a GP-friendly, well-balanced meal plan *might* look like. It's not to be taken as a one-size-fits-all meal plan.

Day 1

Breakfast: Quick & Easy Pancakes (92); Baked Breakfast Sausage (83)

Juice: Berry Good Juice (96)

Lunch: Turkey Soup (120)

Dinner: 3 ounces skinless Roasted Chicken & 3/4 cup Root Vegetables (124)

Smoothie: Go-To Green Smoothie (99)

Day 2

Breakfast: Pumpkin Spice Quinoa & Rice (82)

Juice: Grapes & Greens Juice (97)

Lunch: 1-1/2 cups Chicken & Root Vegetable Soup (116)

Dinner: 4 ounces 10-Minute Salmon (132); 3/4 cup Carrot Ginger Bisque (119)

Smoothie: Pina Colada Smoothie (102)

Day 3

Breakfast: Spinach & Egg Casserole (85)

Juice: Carrot Ginger Juice (95)

Lunch: 1-1/2 cups Chicken Noodle Soup (121)

Dinner: Tomato-Less Meatloaf (131); 1/2 cup Creamy Mashed Potatoes (144)

Smoothie: Almond Joy Smoothie (105)

Day 4

Breakfast: Turkey & Carrot Hash (87)

Juice: Daily Green Juice (94)

Lunch: Bison Stew (129)

Dinner: Tilapia Florentine (134); 1/2 cup Basic Quinoa (147)

Smoothie: Sweet-Banana Smoothie (105)

Eating in Restaurants

Eating in restaurants while following a GP-friendly diet can be challenging, but it's certainly doable. The key is being proactive and having a plan.

Choose the restaurant

Become familiar with restaurants in your area that either offer GP-friendly options or are willing to adapt menu items to suit your needs. Whenever possible, suggest one of these restaurants when choosing where to eat.

Steakhouses and seafood restaurants tend to work well as they typically offer grilled or baked poultry and fish, as well as potatoes, steamed vegetables, and rice. Italian restaurants and Mexican restaurants can be trickier, as many dishes contain high-fat and/or high-fiber ingredients like cheese, sauces, and beans. "Bar food" menus tend to be difficult to adapt as much of it is fried food.

Call ahead

If you're going out to eat for a special occasion, such as a birthday, anniversary, or graduation, consider calling ahead to explain your dietary restrictions and requests. This tends to work best with small or independent restaurants rather than larger chain restaurants. You may be able to talk directly to the chef and work with him or her to develop a meal that will be both appropriate for your needs and enjoyable to your palate.

Be sure you know what you're requesting before you call. Be specific yet flexible and see what he or she can do. For example, "Would it be possible to get a grilled chicken breast or piece of fish, using only the minimal amount of oil necessary, with a plain baked potato or sweet potato, and a side of well-steamed veggies like carrots or peas, again with as little added fat as possible?"

Know what you're going to order before you arrive

It can be uncomfortable to search a menu for GP-friendly items while others look on, asking whether or not there's anything you can eat.

The good news is almost all chain restaurants and many independent establishments now post their menus online. Some also provide nutrition information, which is extremely valuable since seemingly healthy dishes can sometimes be loaded with fat. If possible, do your research ahead of time and decide what you're going to order so that you don't even have to open the menu. Always have a second choice, just in case!

Ask for what you want

Order what you want, whether that means just a side dish or something off of the children's menu. Also, don't be afraid to make simple modifications, such as no sauce or hold the cheese, or basic special requests. Even if it's not on the menu, you can almost always get a plain grilled chicken breast and a baked potato, for example. Be polite, of course, and if necessary explain very simply that you have dietary restrictions due to a health condition.

Enjoy the company

Do your best to focus your attention on the people you're with and the conversation taking place rather than the food. While that's certainly easier said than done, being social and continuing to spend time with friends – even if that means watching other people eat food that you wish you could be eating – is usually better for the spirit than sitting at home alone.

If you find this especially difficult, try suggesting activities that involve food but do not revolve around food. Bowling, festivals, and sporting events are good examples. Our local comedy club serves dinner during the show. It's bar food so I bring my own meal, but nobody's focus is on the food, it's on the stage. I've heard of movie theaters that are serving dinner now, as well. Do some research and be creative!

Attending Parties & Celebrations

Like eating in restaurants, eating at others' houses and attending parties and holiday events can seem nearly impossible in the context of a gastroparesis-friendly diet. The truth is, it *is* possible to not just attend social gatherings but to actually enjoy them. Again, the key is to plan ahead and be your own advocate throughout every step of the process.

Be Choosy

Don't accept every invitation you receive. Prioritize the ones that are most important to you, where you will most enjoy the company and feel most comfortable. All of these factors will affect how you feel physically and your ability to enjoy yourself despite the limitations of a GP-friendly diet.

Be Honest

Talk with the host ahead of time and let him or her know about your current situation. Simply explain that you have a medical condition that requires a strict diet. Depending on your relationship, you may choose to go into more or less detail. Let them know that you will be bringing your own food (see below), not because you don't want to eat what they are preparing but because you want to feel well and be able to enjoy the company.

When you accept the invitation, do let the host know that your symptoms are sometimes unpredictable, despite adherence to your special diet, and there's a small possibility that you may not be able to attend. Unless you feel absolutely awful, however, I recommend following through on your plan. Sometimes getting out, socializing, and talking about things other than gastroparesis can do wonders for the spirit if not the body.

Bring Your Own Food

I recommend always bringing your own food. If it's a plated dinner, arrange with the host to serve the food that you've prepared. You might even ask what they are serving and make your own GP-friendly version. Otherwise, simply bring whatever you'd ordinarily eat for a meal. If something else is served that happens to be GP-friendly, by all means partake and enjoy!

Others in attendance may not even notice that your meal is different and those who do will likely understand with a simple explanation that you have special dietary needs. Try to promptly and politely change the subject if you do not wish to draw attention to your meal and your medical condition. In general, the less awkward you feel, the less likely others are to notice.

Potlucks and buffet meals are even easier. Simply bring a GP-friendly dish or two. There may be other things you can eat as well, but if not you know you'll have at least one or two safe dishes to enjoy.

If you will not be bringing your own food, always eat before you go. The worst-case scenario is to show up hungry, without any of your own food, and find that there's nothing GP-friendly for you to eat.

Avoid Alcohol

Alcohol is a known gastric irritant. It can also delay gastric emptying, especially when combined with a high-fat meal. Some people with gastroparesis are able to tolerate small amounts of alcohol, but most find that they are able to better manage their symptoms while abstaining with alcohol. If you do choose to drink alcohol and are maintaining a low-FODMAP or gluten-free diet, keep in mind that beer and grain alcohol often contains gluten.

Change Your Focus

The more you can focus on the company and conversation, the less you will fixate on the food and the more fun these kinds of events will be. Easier said than done, I know, but by following the guidelines above you'll set yourself up to have a good time and feel as well as possible.

Maintaining a Healthy Weight

It's common for those diagnosed with gastroparesis to lose weight, often a significant amount, due to a combination of severe symptoms and a restrictive diet. It's also common, however, for people to gain weight after a GP diagnosis for these very same reasons.

As counter intuitive as it seems, the same tips apply to gaining and losing weight. For most people it has less to do with the amount of calories consumed and more to do with the source of those calories and the availability of nutrients that regulate hormones and metabolism. Whether you're unintentionally losing weight or gaining weight, these mechanisms are not functioning properly. Focusing on the *quality* of the food in your diet is the first step to maintaining a healthy weight, while also improving your overall health and reducing GP symptoms.

Get more "bang for your bite"

Swap white, processed, and/or refined foods for more colorful, nutrient-rich foods as suggested throughout this book. Foods that provide calories but do not nourish your body will not help with long-term weight maintenance.

Eat more fat

While a gastroparesis-friendly diet should be low in dietary fat, it is possible to restrict fat too much, making weight management quite difficult. Dietary fat is essential for regulation of the hormones that control appetite and metabolism, as well as the absorption of the fat-soluble vitamins, A, D, E, and K.

Stop snacking

While you may think that frequent snacking, also called grazing, is the best way to pack in calories, it may actually be working against you. First, GP-friendly "snacks" aren't usually well-balanced. They tend to be mostly empty carbs with little nutritional value. Second, continuous snacking never allows your stomach to make any progress with digestion. Continuous snacking may exacerbate symptoms, especially fullness, nausea, bloating, and pain in the afternoon and evening. This often results in skipping evening meals or even breakfast the next day, leading to even poorer nutrition.

Drink responsibly

Many GPers rely on liquid calories to help with weight maintenance. If you're drinking soda or sports drinks, however, these empty calories are not nourishing the body and may be contributing to worsening gut health and blood sugar dysregulation. This may make it more difficult to gain weight.

On the flip side, if you are consuming diet drinks in an effort to lose weight, keep in mind that artificial sweeteners often exacerbate gastrointestinal symptoms and have been found to increase appetite, stimulate sugar cravings, and cause hypoglycemia, making *weight loss* more difficult.

Be comprehensive

Dietary modifications are not and should not be the only means of managing symptoms, nor are they the only considerations for weight maintenance. Mild to moderate physical activity can be very helpful, though it has nothing to do with calorie burn. Exercise can alleviate digestive symptoms, which may allow you to eat more well-balanced, nourishing meals. It also helps to lower stress levels and promote restful sleep, both of which play important roles in weight maintenance. If you are not sleeping well and/or feel very stressed or anxious (whether about your symptoms, your weight, or other challenges in your life), that may be a bigger factor in your weight struggles than your diet. The good news is that a comprehensive gastroparesis management plan covers all of these areas and will likely help address your weight struggles, as well as symptom management.

Following a Vegetarian or Vegan Diet

There are many restrictions within the gastroparesis-friendly diet itself and adding more parameters can quickly become overwhelming and/or nutritionally unsound. For this reason, I generally caution against following a vegan diet, at least immediately after diagnosis.

That said, I know there are ethical and religious reasons that play into these choices and I do believe that with extra planning, support, and diligence, it can be possible for those with gastroparesis to safely follow a strict vegetarian and even vegan diet. As with other dietary approaches, the key is to implement the guidelines *within* the context of a gastroparesis-friendly diet.

Fiber

Nutrient-rich plant-based diets tend to be high in fiber due to high consumption of grains, fruits, vegetables, nuts, seeds, and legumes. It's important to modify and tailor your food choices to suit gastroparesis management.

For example:

- Soak whole grains such as quinoa, millet, and buckwheat prior to cooking to make them easier to digest.
- Choose white rice over brown rice.
- Choose and prepare fruits and vegetables according to GP-friendly guidelines outlined throughout this book.
- Avoid beans and foods with indigestible parts, such as broccoli, popcorn, whole nuts, chia seeds, etc.

Protein

Many plant-based diets emphasize high-fiber sources of plant based proteins, such as legumes. It's important to find lower-fiber sources of plant-based proteins that do not exacerbate symptoms, without relying too heavily on processed foods like protein bars and powders.

Some whole grains, including quinoa, are fairly high in protein. Other sources of GP-friendly, plant-based protein include nut and seeds butters and traditionally-fermented forms of soy, such as miso, natto, and tempeh.

Depending on how strictly you adhere to the vegetarian diet, fish and eggs can be an excellent source of protein, high-quality fat, and other nutrients. This may alleviate the need for supplement proteins in the forms of bars or powders.

Fat

Plant-based fats, such as olive, coconut, and red palm oil, tend to be well-tolerated in small amounts as part of a gastroparesis-friendly diet.

Supplementation

Supplementation will likely be necessary to ensure adequate nutrition given these additional dietary restrictions. A vitamin B12 supplement is typically suggested for all vegetarians and vegans, and a multi-vitamin is recommended for nearly everyone who follows a gastroparesis diet. You may need to experiment to find the supplement(s) that work best for you.

Support

Implementing a nutrient-rich, plant-based, gastroparesis-friendly diet is not easy. I strongly suggest that you consult a qualified nutrition professional to help you design your own plan based on your tolerances and goals. Most nutrition professionals are not familiar with gastroparesis, so I encourage you to bring this book and work with them to ensure that all of your needs are met.

Additional Resources & Guidance

It is my sincerest hope that what you've read in this book has left you feeling empowered and inspired as you begin to implement your own nutrient-rich, GP-friendly diet. Please be mindful that dietary choices are only one part of an effective gastroparesis management plan.

You'll find hundreds of blog posts, videos, and free classes focused on helping you learn to live well (or get well!) with gastroparesis on my website (www.LivingWithGastroparesis.com). I've also created the following resources to help you on your journey:

Quick-Start Guide to Gastroparesis Management

The Quick Start Guide to Gastroparesis Management was created to put you on the path to improved symptom management and a better quality of life *right now*. In this 40-page eBook, I take you step-by-step through the most effective changes you can make to start feeling better ASAP. If you're newly diagnosed and/or completely overwhelmed, this is an ideal place to start.

For more information or to purchase a copy, visit: http://bit.ly/gpquickstart.

Living (Well!) with Gastroparesis

Living (Well!) with Gastroparesis: Answers & Advice for a Healthier, Happier Life covers all areas of the comprehensive gastroparesis management plan in an easy-to-understand Q&A format. Topics include understanding gastroparesis, becoming your own advocate, appropriate medical treatment, complementary therapies, dietary modification, nutrition, supplementation, lifestyle practices, stress management, socializing, relationships, coping skills, and more.

Read the first chapter for free or purchase in paperback or Kindle format at: http://amzn.to/gastroparesisbook.

Living (Well!) with Gastroparesis: Self-Guided Program

The Living (Well!) with Gastroparesis Self-Guided Program is the most comprehensive resource I've created to date, consisting of 12 mp3 classes and dozens of worksheets and handouts, covering all aspects of living (well!) with gastroparesis. It's everything I'd tell you if we could sit down together and walk through your personalized management plan, step by step, trouble-shooting the challenges that come up along the way.

Coming October 2014. To learn more, visit: http://www.gastroparesisprogram.com.

ABOUT THE AUTHOR

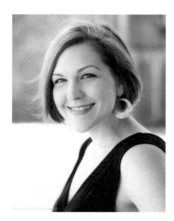

Crystal Zaborowski Saltrelli is a speaker, author, and Certified Health Coach. With her books, classes, videos, and website, Crystal has helped thousands of people worldwide learn to live (well!) with gastroparesis.

Crystal's interest in holistic health and nutrition began soon after she was diagnosed with idiopathic gastroparesis in 2004 at the age of 23. She went on to study Health Counseling and Holistic Nutrition at the Institute for Integrative Nutrition and became certified by the American Association of Drugless Practitioners in 2010. She also has a Bachelor's Degree from Dartmouth College and has completed continuing education coursework via the Harvard School of Medicine.

Crystal is the author of two books, *Eating for Gastroparesis* and *Living (Well!) with Gastroparesis*,. Crystal also serves as Nutritional Specialist for the Gastroparesis & Dysmotilities Foundation and is a patient-advocate for the Digestive Health Alliance.

Crystal lives in upstate New York with her husband and their two-year-old daughter. For more information about living well with gastroparesis or to contact Crystal, please visit her website at www.CrystalSaltrelli.com.